MEDICINE MADAMS
AND MOUNTIES

Medicine Madams and Mounties

Stories of a Yukon Doctor
1933–1947

Allan Duncan

RAINCOAST BOOKS

Vancouver

First published in 1989 by
Raincoast Book Distribution Ltd.
112 East 3rd Avenue
Vancouver, BC   V5T 1C8

Reprinted 1994

CANADIAN CATALOGUING IN PUBLICATION DATA

Duncan, Allan C., 1908–
Medicine Madams and Mounties: Stories of a Yukon Doctor

ISBN 0-920417-67-1

1. Duncan, Allan C., 1908– 2. Physicians – Yukon Territory – Biography
3. Yukon Territory – Biography   I. Title.

FC 4023.1.D39A3 1989   971.9 102 0924   C89-091225-4   F109.D39 1989

Cover design by Trina Owen/Map by Nick Murphy
Typesetting by Mediaworks

Printed in Canada

Dedicated to my loving family

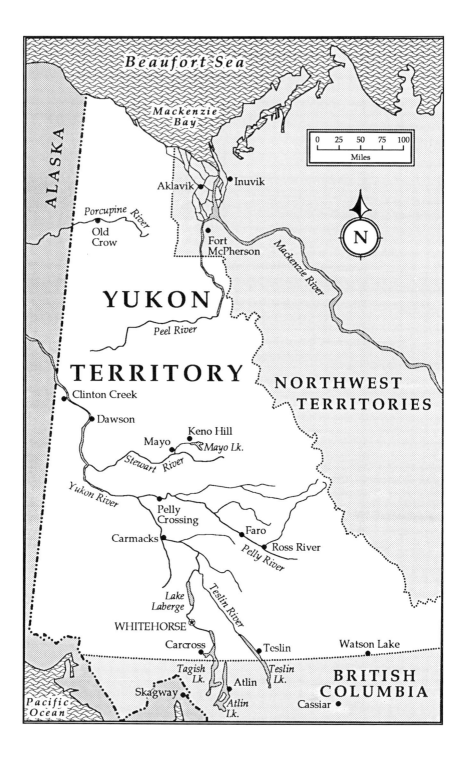

CONTENTS

Author's note

When I went to the Yukon as a young doctor in 1933 the practice of medicine had hardly changed since the days of the Gold Rush. The isolation, scanty population and poverty of the territory had effectively cut off the people of the Yukon from the advances taken for granted in the South. When I left, 14 years later, after the war, the medical care was as good as any in Canada. I was present, then, during a time of rapid change in the practice and science of medicine.

A doctor in the Yukon in those days had to work by himself, often far away from a hospital and with virtually no chance of getting any expert help or advice. Emergencies had to be tackled with the equipment that could be carried with him. He had to be internist, orthopaedic surgeon, obstetrician, dentist and even detective to help the RCMP. And all this in a climate that made even the simplest tasks difficult!

My years as a doctor in the Yukon were times of great satisfaction when I managed to cheat death and even greater disappointment when I failed. And I must confess that often I was very afraid: afraid of dying because there was no other doctor to treat me if I was ill or injured; and afraid of dying from drowning, airplane crashes and exposure in the bush as I went out to treat my patients in their cabins and camps. Thank God for the many friends and helpers who were there when I needed them!

My only regret is that my long hours of work and absences from home meant that I did not have much free time to spend with my wife and three sons.

I hope they understood.

Introduction

To read this book is, for me, like attending a reunion of old friends; I knew almost everybody in these pages – from Irving Snider, who filled my teeth in the summertime, to my own father, who filled my teeth in the winter when the town was without a dentist. I didn't know Ruby, Dawson's most famous madam, whose little building is now a heritage building, but I knew *of* her. And I knew poor Dr. Nunn, who suffered a burst appendix and, because there was no other doctor in town, faced certain death unflinchingly.

Dr. Duncan's book is an important work of social history but, unlike some dry-as-dust volumes, it is never less than lively. A doctor views the world from an odd perspective; he also sees and notes all manner of strange and curious incidents which the average journalist or historian can never capture. The author is fortunate in having a retentive memory, an eye for anecdote, and a wry sense of humour. But his greatest fortune has been to preside over some of the most fascinating patients any medical man was blessed with, at a moment in history that can never be recaptured.

The Yukon in the Thirties was unique. It resembled no other corner of Canada – indeed no other corner of the world. Dr. Duncan saw it all, and it is a service to his readers as well as future historians that he has made this vanished era come alive.

– *Pierre Berton*

PROLOGUE

Heading due North

On the way to the Yukon

One night soon after I had arrived in the Yukon I saw a tall, lithe man coming down the road toward my log cabin. The moon was full. The man walked strangely, gliding over the ground like a boxer stalking an opponent, tilting slightly, moving on his toes. On his head was a leather cap. Under his long coat he wore moose-skin mukluks.

The man knocked on my door. A patient, I thought, and let him in. He introduced himself as George Ortell, a fur trapper and prospector, and then got straight to the point: "Do you know how to start a fire in the bush without matches?"

The problem was far from my mind. My cabin was warm and snug but I told him I'd be interested in his solution. Ortell took off his cap. He had cut the stitches that joined the pie-shaped segments, leaving only the button at the top to hold the pieces together. I couldn't resist asking about the gaps between the flaps. He replied that the 'ventilation' was to keep his brain cool. Since he was almost bald I thought he must be some kind of lunatic.

Ortell asked me for a 30.30 shell. I reluctantly gave him one.

With some twists of his massive fingers, and a little help from his teeth, he removed the bullet from the casing and then packed the empty space left above the cordite with bits of lint and wool collected from my jacket and his shaggy woollen coat. He went out to the wood shed, brought back some firewood and a handful of twigs and piled the wood teepee-fashion on the kitchen floor. Next, he took my rifle from the wall rack, inserted the bullet-less shell and before I could protest took aim at the pile of wood and fired. The cordite explosion ignited the lint and the burning lint set the twigs on fire. I started to put the fire out and when I looked up Ortell had silently slipped out into the darkness.

Much later, after we had become friends, I came to understand why he had come to my cabin that night. He had heard there was a new doctor in Mayo, someone who had never been to the North before, and it occurred to him that like everyone else in the Arctic I had to learn how to survive. It certainly wasn't the kind of welcome I had anticipated when I had left Winnipeg a few weeks before.

Only doctor for 400 miles

On a spring day earlier that year the medical superintendent at the Winnipeg General Hospital called me to his office and said that a mining firm in a place called Stewart, north of Vancouver, needed a doctor to look after its workers. The pay was $250 a month with a house thrown in. I was twenty-four and almost broke. The salary and free house seemed a godsend and I wasn't the least bit concerned by the fact that I'd be the only doctor for 400 miles.

I found Stewart on the map—a tiny dot north of Prince Rupert, near the B.C.-Alaska border. I borrowed some money to buy a trunk and a raincoat, bought my rail ticket to Vancouver and said good-bye to all my friends at the hospital. When I got to Winnipeg station I found Archbishop Stringer and his wife were waiting to see me off. He was wearing his full clerical regalia and his wife had baked some cookies for me. At first I was too shy to admit that I didn't have the vaguest idea what they were doing there. Then, as we were talking, the Archbishop explained that his archdiocese included the Yukon. "So what are you doing here?" I asked. Gently, he pointed out that I was going to the mining town of Mayo, on the banks of the Stewart River, in the Yukon.

My next surprise was my reception at Vancouver. A nurse I knew in Winnipeg had asked her father, a clergyman, and her brother to meet me at the CN station. We went to their home where I was to spend the day before embarking on the steamer *Norah* for Skagway. The brother almost proved to be my undoing, for he gave me a glass of his homemade wine and then another and then another. I had hardly touched alcohol until then but I did not wish to appear unappreciative. After a few more glasses I was enjoying a pleasant stupor. Luckily his father kept track of the time, loaded me into his car and delivered me to the *Norah*'s gangplank just in time. "My boy," said the minister, as he pushed me up the gang plank, "give the purser your ticket and go straight to your cabin. See and talk to nobody—absolutely nobody."

Later I remembered noticing that the ship's guard rails were crowded with people watching me board the ship. Old people, young people, children, and a few pregnant women; all curious to see the new doctor who was destined to attend them for a year. The next morning I peered out of the porthole and was treated to a magnificent sight: a panorama of bright sunlight on beautiful trees, islands and water. We were gliding along the inside passage to Alaska. Soon the *Norah* was docking at Skagway and from there I rode the White Pass and Yukon Railway to Whitehorse. I checked in at the Whitehorse Inn to await the departure of the first downstream steamer for Mayo and Dawson. I got to know a few of my future fellow travellers; they were all, like me, waiting for the steamer that would take them into the cold land that would be our prison for nearly a year. In those times there was no regular air service and once the Arctic winter arrived we would be trapped.

In a few days our paddle-wheeled steamer, the *Keno*, was ready for passengers. As I had almost missed the *Norah* in Vancouver, I was on the Whitehorse dock long before the *Keno* was due to leave and watched in amazement as she cast her lines and, with her barge lashed to her bow, started to move upstream—south, not north. The *Keno* was not leaving without me, come hell or high water, and as the barge passed I jumped aboard, landing beside a pile of frozen meat. The captain and crew were a little surprised for they were just moving upstream to a wide part of the river where they turned around and tied up again at the dock facing downstream. Then the other passengers and baggage came aboard and the *Keno*, named after the mining town north of Mayo, started off down-river. She was to take us down the Yukon to Stewart, a small settlement at the junction of the Yukon and Stewart Rivers, and from there we would chug up the Stewart for a hundred miles or so to Mayo.

On the good ship Keno

The *Keno* was smaller than the other stern-wheelers plying the Yukon rivers because she had to navigate the Stewart, a shallow river plagued by sand-bars. Old-timers used to say that her skipper, Bill Bromley, could get her to float on a heavy dew. This was the ship that was to be my home for the next three weeks. Pushing a heavily laden barge, the *Keno* made good time down the river swollen with the spring run-off. On our first day out Captain Bromley pointed to a large sand bar covered with trees and told us that it was called Scatter Ass Bar because a group of prostitutes were marooned there for a few days during the gold rush. Then we left the swift-flowing river and steamed into ice-covered Lake Laberge. After a few hours it was clear that forcing our way through the thick ice was going to be a tough job. In those days

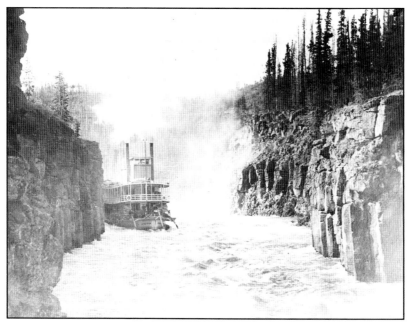

Steamer Sir Clifford Sifton in Miles Canyon

workmen from the shipping company used to put tons of lamp black on the ice along the steamers' course. This black material attracted the sun's heat, melting and making a passage through the ice. We followed this black icy road, pushing into the pack, then backing, then ramming into the pack again. But after a few hours of this we were stuck in the lee of a large island in the centre of the lake.

Since we were obviously going nowhere for several days, I had time to climb to the top of the island's small mountain. When I got back to the *Keno* the crew members told me, with just a hint of a smile, that the bears that I had seen were usually quite hungry in the spring! One day the resident Indian chief, Jim Boss, came on board to sell lake trout the tribe had caught. In the summer season, to amuse the tourists, he used to board the ship to demand a toll from the captain, for permission to cross "his" lake!

After three days the ice was obviously weaker and so we started to crash our way through again. We could not wait any longer because the *Keno* was making the first run of the season and the other steamers were waiting at Whitehorse for us to punch their way through for them. Finally we got out of the lake and into a section of the Yukon called the Thirty Mile - a stretch of wild water, rocks, and shoals and the scene of many wrecks.

Thirty passengers—all going, like me, to Mayo—were on the *Keno* as she started to run the Thirty Mile and, except for me, they all found something to take their minds off the raging river. Among them was Jim Fairborn, a hearty, stout man who was the White Pass agent in Mayo. He kept busy copying invoices with a large jelly duplicator. The first Xerox? When not at work copying Jim played bridge with other passengers in the forward lounge.

At each bend in the river the paddle-wheel was put in reverse. This freed the barge a little and, following the current, it led the *Keno* around the bend. When the bend was sharp the crew gave the barge a little help by tightening and loosening the cables that held it to the prow of the *Keno*. This made the barge pivot to starboard or port, leading the *Keno* around the rocks. I was fascinated and frightened by this technique and as the steamer came to really sharp bends I went on deck, looking ahead and hanging onto the nearest stanchion, while the rest of the passengers kept playing bridge. Fairborn and others kept telling me to sit down and relax but I paid no attention to them. Then, as the *Keno* rounded one bend, I saw that a boulder the size of a small house lay straight ahead. Grasping my stanchion, I yelled, "Hang on!" "Sit down and keep quiet," somebody replied.

Shipwreck

Somehow the man at the winch managed to turn the barge into the rock instead of away from it. With a grinding crash the barge's bow struck the rock, climbing up its inclined surface until it tumbled off to one side. Cargo spilled all over the place. Carcasses of frozen meat slipped into the water. Boxes floated off downstream and heavier pieces of cargo sunk to the river bottom. With the barge stuck fast, the spring current started to push the steamer's

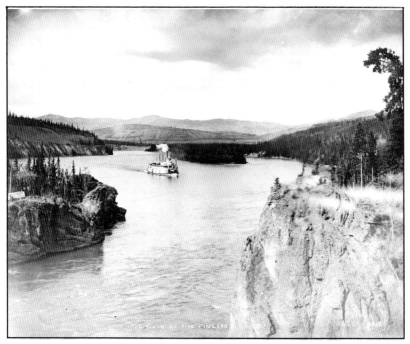

The Yukon tackles the Five Fingers rapids

stern around, damming the river. As a result the water piled up against the *Keno*'s exposed side and pushed her broadside downstream. Her stern struck the opposite bank and her paddle-wheel was ripped off. This freed the steamer which pulled the barge off the rock and soon the whole outfit was drifting, powerless and rudderless, down the raging river.

Nobody on board was seriously hurt and as we drifted down the river the crew tried to run lines ashore to stop the ship. But the steel cables snapped like violin strings and the crewmen who had taken

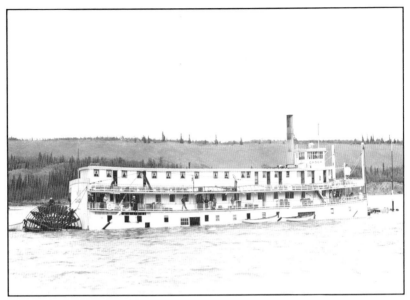

Grounded steamer: ready for salvage

the cables ashore in small boats were marooned. Soon there were so few deckhands that the cook and I had to man the steam-winch controlling the cables holding the barge which was now sinking at the bow, dragging bottom at times. But I could not understand the captain's orders. He would yell "Slacken away on the port!" and I did not know whether that meant I should loosen or tighten the pulleys. Which was port? Right or left? Finally both steamer and barge ran aground on a sand bar at the mouth of the Hootalinqua River. Most of the barge was now under water but the *Keno* was in good shape—except for her smashed paddle and her main and "monkey" rudders, the ones at the extreme stern where they catch the paddle's slipstream.

A few days later another steamer, the *Casca*, arrived from Whitehorse with spare parts and tools. Soon the crews had repaired our paddle wheel and rudders and refloated the barge. For days, however, all sorts of wrecked cargo, clothing, lumber, hats, and baggage floated down the river and that summer many Indian women at Dawson were wearing the latest fashions that came from our wreck. Then we chugged down to Dawson for more permanent work on the barge and came back up the Yukon to Stewart and turned into the Stewart river. Flocks of newly-returned ducks, geese and cranes were everywhere and on the hills black bears were dozing in the sun. We could see moose on the sandbars, feeding on early willow and poplar buds.

Our arrival in Mayo was a gala occasion. Blowing its whistle loudly, the *Keno* rounded the final bend and the town's population was on the dock to greet us. After all, we carried the first fresh food they had seen since the previous September. Almost the instant the ship docked longshoremen began unloading its cargo of canned goods, liquor and heavy equipment and then began loading it and the empty barge with hundreds of tons of silver-lead ore concentrate which had been packed in sacks on the docks during the winter.

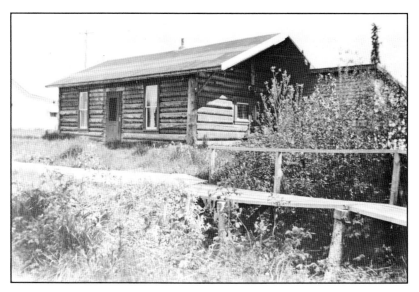

My house and office in Mayo

My job was to relieve Dr. Gordon Ferguson, who had been in Mayo several years. After greeting me at the dock, he took me to the hospital and I was introduced to Alma Jones, matron, general manager, anaesthetist and all-round good nurse, and her assistant, Lillian Ross. Bill Bromley was also visiting friends in the hospital with one of his crew, Chuck Beaumont. The two men were always playing practical tricks on the nurses. But Miss Jones had her revenge when she gave Bromley some gum containing a laxative and the poor man had to spend most of the journey back to Whitehorse running up and down the steps from his wheelhouse to the toilet on the main deck.

Dr. Ferguson and his wife sailed on the Keno the day after I arrived. I watched them go and realized that although I was excited by the prospect of having my own medical practice I was also worried about whether I could survive in this vast, strange and somewhat foreboding land.

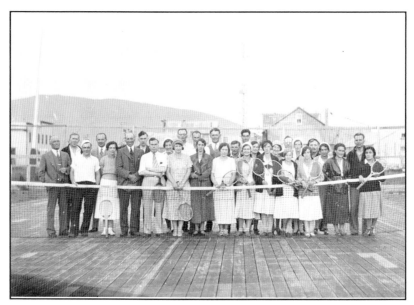

Midnight tennis party in Mayo.

PART ONE

MAYO

At home and on the dance floor

My home in Mayo was a large log cabin with a big living room and a small office tacked on. There were two large bedrooms. I used one and the big Manx cat, Bugs, who came with the cabin, used the other. He ate his rabbits in this room, batting the bones about at night when he was not out hunting, fighting or fornicating. The kitchen was very large with a long-handled pump fixed, not in a sink, but in the middle of a massive, immovable bench. The pump had to be primed, for it tapped a water table deep in the permafrost and, of course, it froze solid in the winter and I had to buy water.

Like most buildings in the Yukon, my cabin had ventilators—holes about eight inches in diameter drilled high in the walls and lined with short pieces of stove pipe and dampers. To close or open the ventilator you pulled on a cord that raised the flap. I could never find out why ventilation was such a fetish in the north. There was enough natural ventilation through chinks in the walls of cabins and houses. And nearly all doors had been heaved by permafrost and so fitted badly. Whatever the reason, all rooms had

15

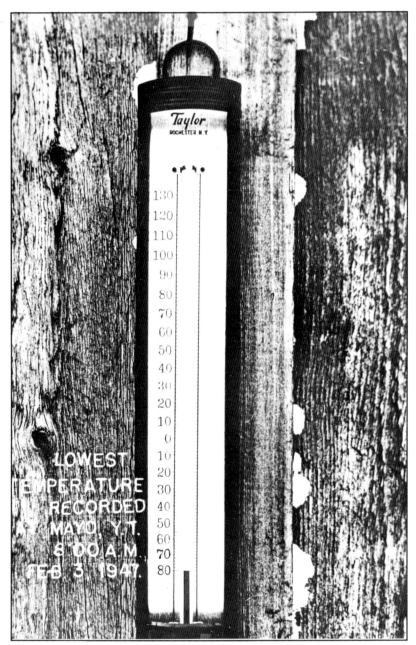

Coldest recorded temperature in Yukon.
Photograph by Gordon McIntyre

to have these ventilators and although they had wire screens on the outside, flies, mosquitoes and spiders found them convenient runways into the homes.

Heat was provided by "Yukon Heaters" - oval-shaped metal drums on legs. A stove pipe ran straight up through the roof, protected by an outer pipe called a "safety." An airspace between the two pipes insulated the roof from the hot pipe. Three of these heaters tried to warm my cabin but water in a pail still froze every night in the winter. The cold gradually crept up from the floor to the ceiling as the night wore on and so a quick glance at the cat's position in the morning would give me the room temperature. If Bugs was sleeping on the piano top, rather than on the floor, it was very cold. The key-hole test was another way to tell winter temperature. The cold air flowing through the key-hole produced a vapor trail into the room and its length measured the outside frost level. Yet another indication of the outside temperature could be seen in the bathroom. The nail heads on the inside sheathing carried the frost into the room and this produced beautiful glistening buttons on the studs; the bigger the buttons the colder it was outside.

Our electricity came from a large diesel generator. Power was available from early morning until eleven thirty at night unless some special event, such as a dance, called for later service. About twenty minutes before black-out the generator's operator would flick the power off for a second. This brought all bridge, poker, and other social events such as dances to an end.

Mayo dances were real community affairs and virtually everybody came. They were held in a hall about four log-lengths long. A log-length was sixteen feet—as long as straight sections could be found in our sub-arctic spruce. At the main entrance there was a large room with a separate heater reserved as a place to leave sleeping babies and for the women to take off the extra underclothes they wore to get to the dance in the 50 to 60 below weather.

The main hall had a long bench running down each side and Mayo convention dictated that the women sit on the right side and the men on the left. The band played on a platform at the far end.

When the music struck up, the men made for the women in a massive wave. There was no way a man could get the partner he wanted unless he made an unseemly dash to his lady friend, but this would be noticed by everyone and recorded as "special" interest. No woman refused a dance invitation, unless the man was drunk or obviously undesirable. Men outnumbered women two to one so there were no female wall-flowers. This meant that the married men could nip out for a drink while their wives danced. Music in Mayo was excellent, largely because of the skill of Sergeant Claude Tidd, RCMP Tidd's favorite instrument was the slide trombone, but he played anything that could be blown, stroked or beaten. He could hear a new tune on the radio and, presto, it was on the program for the next dance. The man who ran the light plant kept the diesel going a few extra hours on dance nights but around one in the morning the huge drum heaters were doused and all water was drained from taps. Then, just before the lights went out, the babies were collected, long bloomers put on and everyone went home to bed.

Wolves don't attack people, do they?

The hall was used for other social functions, such as the Mayo Anglican Women's Auxiliary annual dinner, and one winter night when a bone-chilling wind swept through town, I went to the hall expecting a good meal and some pleasant female company. As I took off my coat, however, the Mountie in charge of the Keno detachment, Corporal Ted McAskill, told me that an old miner named Sanquist had been found unconscious in his cabin at Duncan Creek, about twenty miles out on the road to Keno. I agreed to go with him and McAskill left the hall to pick up Constable Roy Thomas. Then the three of us set off in the old

RCMP car. When we were close to Williams Creek we parked the car in the snow just off the road. From here we had to go down a steep hillside trail to Duncan Creek and could follow the frozen river to Sanquist's cabin.

At first the going was fine. The hard-packed snow was lit by the moon with a bluish green hue and we could find our way easily. Then, as we came to a sharp bend in the creek, I looked up and froze. In the bush were a half dozen pairs of green eyes. Timber wolves. The green eyes moved along, following us a few feet away, until one wolf raised his head and howled right at us. My hair stood up and a tingling raced up and down my spine. I was so scared I nearly wet my trousers. McAskill blithely assured me that wolves never attack people, an assurance that was most welcome but hard to prove. The wolves followed us right to Sanquist's door where they stood on a small hill and watched us go in.

We found Sanquist lying unconscious in bed. His friend had covered him with furs before setting off to call the RCMP. After cleaning him up, we tied him to the mattress. McAskill then shouldered the head end of the mattress and took most of the weight, leaving Thomas and I to carry the corners at Sanquist's feet. The wolves escorted us back to the car. By now Thomas and I were exhausted but McAskill was barely winded. Soon we were back in the Mayo hospital where I admitted Sanquist with a moderately severe hemiplegia (stroke). He was soon up and about.

As I left him in the ward I thought of the friends and the food I had left at the hall. But the hall was dark and so I had to walk home through the frigid streets, a lonely bachelor taking some solace in the fact that at least his cat would be there to greet him.

MEDICINE—
MAYO STYLE

The doctor knows best

On hot summer days the trip down-river to Indian Village, a small collection of log cabins about a mile from Mayo, was usually a routine affair. In the fall or spring, however, the same brief journey was often fraught with danger but since I was the town's only doctor I had to go if there was a medical emergency. One cold October afternoon an Indian came to my cabin to get help for a woman who, he said, had been in labor for three days. He had risked his life crossing the Stewart in a small boat to get me and now I had to go back with him. Cakes of ice, some as large as pianos, were rumbling and crashing down the river. Daylight was fading as we got into his small, home-made boat and, easing into the ice-choked river, headed toward the other shore. The current was so swift that it carried us in a wide arc and I thought we would be swept downstream or, worse, would hit an ice floe. Then the outboard motor's propeller caught in the ice and the motor quit. For what seemed like hours the Indian and I had to row and push against the ice until we hit the far shore.

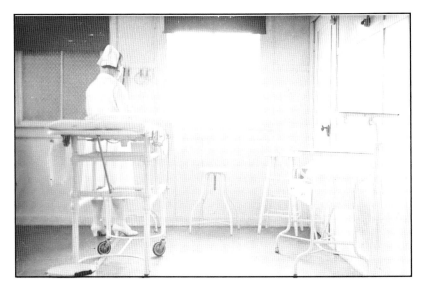

The surgery in Mayo hospital

We walked up the steep bank to a group of cabins surrounded by yapping Indian dogs. These dogs detested the smell of white people and the reverse was equally true. After fighting off the dogs we reached the patient's cabin where some Indian women ushered me into the half-light of a log building. I expected to find the woman on a pile of bedding, probably in a corner. Instead, she was draped face down over a stout pole three feet off the floor. Two women were pulling on her arms and two on her legs to put pressure on her swollen abdomen to force the baby out. The woman, however, had slipped and the pole was across her groin, preventing the baby's head from reaching her pelvic inlet. When my eyes had become accustomed to the dim light, I glanced around the room and saw that the walls were lined by squatting silent Indian women, looking for all the world like a phalanx of Buddhas.

The first thing to do was to find which part of the baby was coming first, head or buttocks. This is always done rectally, never vaginally, because of the danger of infection. As the poor woman was draped over the pole in an inverted U position, a rectal examination was easy but while I was examining her, the woman cursed me continually and the squatting women got up, spat contemptuously on the mud floor and left.

It seemed to me that the baby's head needed to be rotated but, whatever the problem, I could do nothing for the mother in the gloomy, dirty hut. Two men helped me to lift the woman off the pole and put her on an old mattress so that we could take her across the icy river to Mayo hospital. I was not looking forward to the return trip across the river with a patient, but as we were dragging her towards the bank a miracle happened. The woman gave a mighty groan, pushed hard and out popped the baby. It would have been satisfying to say that, with consummate obstetrical skill, I delivered the baby but the birth was so fast and spontaneous that it was all over in about a minute. As we had nothing to tie off the cord with, I used a bit of my shoe-lace and then gave the baby to the Indian women. The Indian and I started home, upstream this time. He freed the boat's propellor, started the engine and worked the boat along the shoreline trying to avoid pieces of ice. Then we crossed the river to Mayo with ice floes rustling and scraping together while a full moon bathed us in pallid light. As we reached shore I asked him why the Indian women had suddenly shown so much disdain for me. He thought for a while and said, "Women say doctor who thinks baby comes out ass hole no good!"

Lost in the frosty night

The prospect of drowning in an ice-clogged river wasn't the only peril that threatened me as I went out on a call. There was also the danger of taking a wrong turn in the wilderness and becoming hopelessly lost.

Late one fall, just before freeze-up, I was asked to go to Keno to see a sick woman. My friend, Rev. Creighton McCullum, offered to drive me there because he could visit some of his parishioners at the same time. It took us about half a day to drive 50 miles over the crooked, pot-holed road. After attending to the woman (she had pneumonia) it was too late to return to Mayo, so McCullum and I decided to stay the night in the Keno Hotel. There was still some daylight after we had finished dinner— light enough, I thought, to take a walk out of town. It was beautiful. The sun was setting beyond the river and cast a dark green shadow over the McQuesten valley. About half a mile out of town I climbed a small ridge and there below me I could see a moving mass of cariboo, probably about ten thousand animals, moving slowly up the valley. Their horns reflected the setting sun and I could hear the clicking of their hooves against the rocks of the moraine. My whole spine tingled, not because I was cold, but because I was watching one of the wonders of nature, the mass migration of the Old Crow-Porcupine cariboo herd on its annual trek south. I walked up to the herd but the animals ignored me. They were too intent on keeping pace with the others. I could see that some slower ones had been wounded by wolves. Packs of howling wolves and yapping coyotes were following the cariboo herd, ready to attack and kill any who fell far behind. Then I walked up another hill and down into a valley hoping to see more of the animals. When I tried to get my bearings I realized that the lights of Keno had disappeared.

It was dark now and I panicked, for my sense of direction was very poor. I tried to convince myself that the town could not be far away and sat down on a rock to think things over. I remembered all the tales I had heard about people starving or freezing to death while they wandered desperately through the wilderness. After ten minutes or so I decided to climb another hill. I looked around and saw a pinprick of light in the distance, a kerosene lamp burning in a cabin window. Was I relieved! As I walked to the cabin, I started shouting "Hello, hello" so as not to startle whoever was in the cabin. A man came to the door and I recognized him as a friend and patient, Angus McLeod. "What the hell are you doing out here at night, Doc?" he asked. I explained what had happened and he invited me in for supper. He put away his cariboo stew and opened a can of sausages—a special treat he had packed over the hills for just such an occasion—and then he opened a can of butter to fry them in. I can still remember the taste of those sausages fried in butter.

After supper McLeod led me back to Keno and on the way we visited his girl friend, Jessie Stewart, the local telephone operator, for a drink. McLeod walked back to his cabin and the cariboo, wolves and coyotes and I went back to my hotel with kind thoughts about my fellow men.

White-out

A year or so later I was caught in a white-out. A woman and her daughter who lived about a mile from Mayo, on the Keno road, sent word that they were both ill and needed a doctor. I started walking in the early afternoon, wearing full winter gear: a fur hat, heavy coon coat, mukluks, warm trousers, a woollen shirt, sweater, heavy socks and underwear. As I trudged along I noticed that the wind was increasing and that streaming dark grey clouds were filling the sky and casting shadows over the ground.

After treating the women, I started to walk back to Mayo. By now the wind had become a gale with fine snow starting to fill the sky. About halfway home my face was getting burned by the bitterly cold snow. Now I could not see through the opalescent screen of driving snow and the road disappeared in the snowdrifts. I could only hope that I was heading, roughly, in the right direction. I was lucky, for after about half an hour I started to pick up the lights in cabins on each side of the snow-covered road. Now I could see where to walk and I was soon at home in the warm.

How to survive at 60 below

Soon after I arrived in Mayo I realised that if I was to be a good doctor in the Yukon I had to know how to survive white-outs and extreme cold. So I decided to find out how the trappers lived when out on their lines.

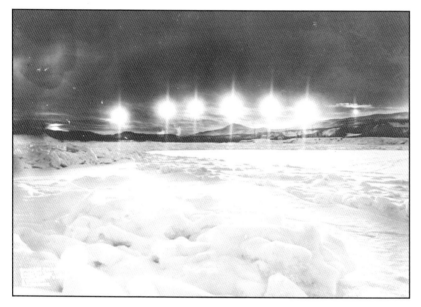

Shortest day: photos shot every 15 minutes

A trapper with a line of a hundred miles or more would build himself several full-sized cabins about twenty to thirty miles apart for sleeping and storing fuel and food. Most trappers also built small "boxes" to protect themselves from the weather if they had to spend a night between their base cabins. These "boxes" were built of logs, about seven to eight feet long, three feet high and three feet wide, with a roof of small logs, topped with plenty of moss. You climbed in through a small opening at one end, just big enough to crawl into comfortably. The door was usually a flap of old canvas.

When night came the trapper tethered his sleigh dogs to trees far enough apart that they could not fight and gave each dog its quota of one dried salmon. Then he crawled into the "box." He warmed up his food and drink on a small Primus stove and then went to sleep inside a heavy sleeping bag with his head close to the canvas flap. Some trappers took a pet sleigh dog, usually a bitch, with them to help keep them warm. The dog also acted as sentinel to warn the trapper if any wolves were around. The trappers always kept a loaded rifle pointing out through the canvas flap, for wolves would attack the tethered dogs and kill them.

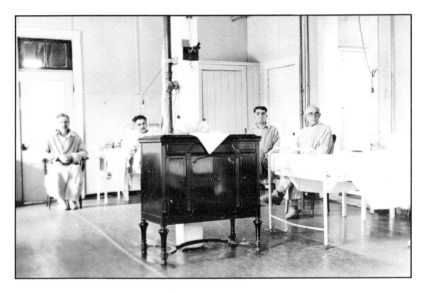

Sitting up: a ward in Mayo hospital

It's fine, doc, but for the whistle

One winter day a husky man with red hair named Gibson drove his dog team up to the Mayo hospital and asked to see me. After he had peeled off his parka he told me that he ran a trap line on the Bonnet Plume River, a tributary of the Peel. "Doc," he said, "I have a big scab in my ear that won't heal. Could you give me some medicine?"

The "scab" was clinically a basal-cell cancer, a slow-growing cancer that does not spread to the rest of the body like other cancers but eats away the adjacent flesh. The only treatment available in Mayo was surgical excision because we hadn't the equipment to give him radiation and Gibson could not afford to go to Edmonton or Vancouver. At first I thought the whole ear should come off but later decided to just do a wide local excision. Gibson agreed. He said he'd like to have some ear left to support his glasses. I removed the growth by cutting away most of the central part of the ear. This created a hole about one and a half inches across but left the top of the ear rim intact. Gibson could wear his glasses and off he went, a happy man.

Next spring, however, he came back. "That damned ear has to got to be fixed," he roared at me. I thought that the cancer had come back. Not so. He was angry because the wind whistled as it blew past the hole in his ear! I noticed that the opening in the ear was almost level with the skin on Gibson's skull. Perhaps his ear was functioning like a flute. I suggested stitching the edges of the hole to a circular incision in the skin just behind his ear. This would, in effect, close up the hole but still allow Gibson the use of that ear. Would Gibson agree? He said, "Yes," and lost his whistling ear.

Later I had another patient with the same disease. This man, a prospector and trapper, had a large ulcer that was eating away his right lower eye-lid. I had to remove the whole lower lid but this, of course, would leave the lower eye-ball unprotected. For days I wondered how to cover it and finally decided that the skin to do the job would have to come from his temple. I cut away the lower eye-lid and made a substitute from the skin on his temple. It healed very well but since it came up over his eye-ball it looked at first as if his eye was peeking over a fence. A few months later the patient came back to see me. His appearance was amazing. The flap, coming from a hairy area, sported a beautiful tuft of hair. It looked like a small pigtail growing beneath his eye! I nicked the flap so that it did not obscure his vision but left his tuft alone and he went away a very satisfied man.

Mauled by a grizzly

One day Cpl. McAskill phoned to tell me that a prospector named Keating had been badly mauled by a grizzly bear. McAskill wanted me to bring a truck, splints and whatever else might be needed. At first I could not get a truck but finally Billy Jeffries, whose father ran the local Taylor and Drury general store, said he would drive one of his father's old delivery trucks to Keno if I guaranteed the gas. I agreed and off we went.

Keating had been prospecting promising ground on Lightning Creek, which runs down a valley from Mount Hinton, when he surprised a grizzly bear with cubs. She was very aggressive and so Keating went to Keno to get help from McAskill. As the two men were walking back up Lightning Creek the grizzly attacked. Keating, in the rear, took the brunt. The bear ripped open his left cheek with one clout, just missing his eye, and then smashed his arm, thigh and knee with the second. By now McAskill had his rifle aimed at the bear but was unable to fire without endangering Keating. Then she charged McAskill. His first shot broke her front leg without slowing her charge but the second hit her in the face and the bear fell dead a few feet in front of him.

McAskill then walked back to Keno and sent the message to me for help. Ten miners and prospectors were waiting in Keno to pack Keating out on a buckboard pulled by a tired-looking horse. Jeffries and I joined them. These men from Keno were as tough a group as you could find but they were afraid of the grizzlies. They would not leave their cabins without a rifle for there were no trees here to give protection from the bears.

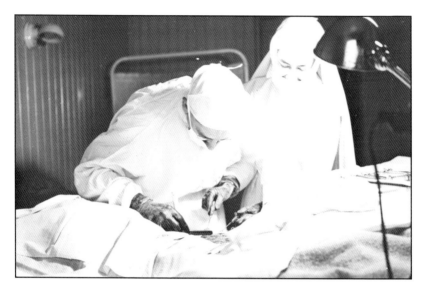

Author at work in surgery

We trudged up Lightning Creek, fighting off the mosquitoes that filled your mouth and nostrils and keeping our eyes open for any more grizzlies. After an hour we reached Keating, guarded by McAskill. Keating was in severe pain and bleeding badly but I thought we could save him for he had no vital injury and, a good sign, was cussing everything and everybody and demanding a drink of whisky. A good slug of morphine worked wonders in a few minutes and we put him on the buckboard and started down the creek to Keno. When the cussing started again, he was given more morphine. At Keno the stretcher was placed in the truck from Mayo and as Billy Jeffries drove, I sat with Keating. It was a long, slow, bumpy ride to the Mayo hospital.

The matron, Alma Jones, with the nurses on duty, Lillian Ross and Jean McCullum, helped me clean up Keating and we dressed his superficial wounds. Keating was now in heavy shock and had lost a lot of blood. We had no blood, no plasma expanders and no antibiotics but we did have our own water replacement - made from melted snow water, filtered and made isotonic by a sodium chloride pill. Of course, the snow had to come from an area where there were no rabbits! This home-made saline solution was given by drip from an enema can. Keating's haemoglobin count was very high, confirming the dehydration and so we gave him several litres of our saline solution and his blood pressure and pulse improved.

The next step was to find a suitable anaesthetic. We usually used open ether, safe but nauseating, slow and a poor relaxant. Our patient, however, was an alcoholic and alcoholics are hard to put to sleep with ether, for alcohol and ether are closely related. And how to hold a mask over his torn face for a long time? I decided to mix one third chloroform with the ether to put him to sleep quickly and then use pure ether administered through a curved tube inserted in his throat. We tackled his face first and took out all the grass and mud. There was a large hole where his cheek should have been but his jaw and most of his teeth were intact and his cheek flap was large so I pulled the flap over and stitched it to the side of his nose.

Then we set his arm and looked at what was left of his thigh and knee. The pieces of his lower thigh were put together and tacked with cat-gut. His knee was not going to work, no matter what we did, because the muscles controlling it were torn. Our chief concern was the possibility of gangrene and tetanus and so we placed rubber drains in almost every cavity and stitched his wounds very loosely. Then we put the whole limb in a cradle-like splint, wrapped adhesive tape around his calf and attached this to a pulley to keep the leg straight.

The result? Minimum shock, no haemorrhage and very little infection, despite the fact that Keating had a bad case of delirium tremens and raved and thrashed about. But when he was well enough to get out of bed we could see that we had to fix his knee for he could put no weight on the injured leg. I decided to fuse the joint, opened the knee, moved the knee-cap to one side and used a small carpenter's saw to square off the ends of the tibia and the shattered knee-joint. The raw surfaces fitted well together but how could I hold them together? I decided to use two four-inch spikes driven criss-cross through the fusion, drilled the holes and inserted the spikes so that they were a snug fit with the ends protruding each side of the joint. Soon the bones knitted and we took out the spikes. Keating's leg was a little short and he limped like Chester in the TV show Gunsmoke but he lived for many years happily drinking his own potent home brew.

Hospital target practice

Late one summer evening a truck drove up to the Mayo hospital. It was Elmer Middlecroft bringing a neighbour, John Darblo, who had been hurt while working a placer claim on Highet Creek. Elmer was driving his horse and rig down the Mayo River road past Darblo's cabin when he decided to visit John. As he walked up to the cabin, he heard a faint voice calling for help. Down in the mining "cut" he found Darblo pinned under a large boulder that had rolled on him when he was digging around it in search of the coarse large gold nuggets often found on the bedrock floor close to large rocks. The boulder had pinned Darblo's leg at the thigh and he had been trapped for nearly 24 hours, yelling for help until Elmer came along. Elmer freed the leg with crowbars. It was a dark purple color, swollen and paralysed. Then Elmer went to his own claim, got his truck and drove Darblo to Mayo.

I often wondered about rescues like this. What prompted Elmer to visit John on this occasion? They met rarely. Was it mental telepathy?

At first we thought Darblo's leg would go gangrenous but fortunately this did not happen. The femoral artery was pinched but enough blood got through so that the leg survived. However, large patches of skin sloughed off and were covered with proud flesh. I had to cover these granulations with split-skin pinch grafts for

most of the fall and winter. At times everybody—Darblo, the
nurses and I—got depressed and discouraged. Enter our hospital
matron, Alma Jones. She decided that Darblo and the other
chronically-ill miners and trappers needed some diversion and
entertainment. Now men like these did not play bridge and they
had no television to watch. The short-wave radio did not work
when the Northern Lights were active. Men like these loved pets
and they loved to shoot. So Miss Jones allowed the patients to keep
two cats that slept in the end-tables beside the bed pans. The
hospital orderly, Shorty Carter, let the cats in and out and everybody enjoyed them. Then Miss Jones went one better; she set up
a shooting gallery for the men. Targets were set up in the grounds
at various distances from a hospital window. The men took turns
with a .22 rifle and a "spotter" recorded their shots.

Just a left-handed dentist

Elmer Middlecroft and his wife lived about a mile from Mayo
on the road to Keno. They both came from the southern States, as
you could tell from their accents and friendliness. Elmer came into
my waiting room one afternoon and said, "Doc, I have a terrible
tooth-ache. Will you yank it for me?" After years of training in
medicine and surgery, I was being asked to be a dentist! I could not
refuse for the poor man was in agony. His swollen, half-opened
jaw showed that he had an abscess as well as a bad tooth.

The guilty tooth was a lower third molar away back in his
mouth. It was set deep in the swollen gums with most of its crown
gone. Medical graduates in my day were given no training in
pulling teeth but I knew where to start. I anaesthetized the jaw with
a mandibular Novocaine block. While waiting for the Novocaine
to take effect I looked at the assortment of dental instruments that
I had inherited. There were forceps that twisted right; others
twisted left; some looked like corkscrews. Then I stood behind my
patient and tried several instruments to see how they would fit

over the tooth. Finally I chose a vicious-looking pair of forceps with one prong on one blade passing between two prongs on the opposite one. I guessed that these forceps were designed to get below what remained of the crown with the prongs passing under the tooth roots. (I later learned that it was called a cow-horn extractor). After cutting down the gum flaps I got a good grip on the tooth. Then I pulled and twisted and then just squeezed as hard as I could and the whole tooth just popped out with not too much jaw bone.

"That didn't hurt a bit, Doc," Middlecroft said, "so I am not going to pay you the five bucks." I would have liked that five dollars for until my monthly pay-cheque arrived cash was scarce. Then he smiled. "Since you did such a good job I am going to give you a gold nugget." He fished into his pocket and brought out a beautiful nugget shaped like a large almond. I took it to Bill Hutchings, the bank manager, and asked him what it was worth. He said it weighed at least two ounces. "So, at $35 an ounce, it's worth about $70, maybe a little less for rock impurities." I never sold the nugget. I had it made into a pendant, which my wife, Jean, still wears.

From then on I did a lot of extractions because our dentists left for the south during winter. Since I was not trained in dentistry I decided not to accept money but took a bottle of rum instead. Most of my dental patients took a slug of my fee as pre-medication and so when the Mayo nurses noticed a tipsy man coming slowly up the long boardwalk to the hospital with a bottle under his arm they got out the dental forceps. The forceps always seemed awkward in my hand and one day I asked a visiting dentist why the forceps were so poorly designed. "They're not," he said, "all your forceps are for a left-handed dentist!"

Murder - Mayo style

Mayo may not have been the wildest place in Canada in the Thirties but it wasn't exactly the tamest. Fights between drunken miners were frequent. Many a tooth was lost, a jaw knocked awry and I was called upon to sew up more than one nasty cut. Murder, though, was practically unheard of. The miners seldom used weapons, preferring to settle disputes with their fists. Late one evening, however, the RCMP asked me to examine a man who had been murdered at the Chateau Mayo. The Chateau contained a restaurant, a beer parlor and about twenty rooms. It was a comfortable spot: it had running water and, what was rare in Mayo, indoor plumbing.

The dead man lay on the bed in an upstairs room. He had obviously been shot while asleep and was a ghastly sight, for his face had been almost completely blown off by a high-powered rifle. No one in the hotel seemed the least bit appalled by what was obviously cold-blooded murder. A man who was standing nearby said to me, "He was a bloody claim-jumper. He had it coming to him."

Eventually a man was charged and chose trial by jury. It was quite short. The accused admitted shooting the man and Judge McAuley sent the jury out. They returned a verdict of "Not Guilty." McAuley was apoplectic.

"How could you reach such a verdict?" he asked. "This is a gross miscarriage of justice."

"Well, your Honor," the foreman replied, "if we say our friend here is guilty you will have him hanged. We feel the claim-jumper got his just punishment. So finding this fellow not guilty is the way things should be."

MAYO PEOPLE

I will never forget that murder; nor will I forget the hundreds of people in Mayo who made life there so exciting and happy. Here are a few words about some of them:

Kitchen comforts

Henrietta and Charles Van Cleaves ran a road house at the junction of the road to Mayo Lake and Keno. It was a nice homey place. "Scharlie," as his wife called him, was a soft-spoken Dutchman with white hair who kept the place warm and ship-shape. Henrietta was an excellent cook but was so heavy that she could hardly move around the kitchen. She made life easier by having a commode built just to the side of the stove. Usually the commode was hidden but, like most doctors, I often caught people in the most inconvenient positions. One morning I was up very early and walked into the kitchen where I saw Henrietta parked on the commode and flipping pancakes at the same time!

The man who saw castles in the sky

Jack Faulkner, a kind old man, was left as watchman at the Wernecke mine when operations were closed down in 1933. He lived in a cabin on a hill with a view over the McQuesten flats and after visiting patients in Keno I used to visit him and watch for moose and cariboo. Beyond the McQuesten River were the snow-capped Ogilvie Mountains. I often saw mirages over these mountains, visions of sun-drenched medieval-type castles with turrets, moats and towers. They shimmered a few minutes then disappeared and reappeared in a new form. For a long time I never mentioned these visions for fear that I would be laughed at. Finally I told Faulkner about them. He had seen them and so had others. He was surprised, though, that nobody had ever told me that they were reflections of English castles off the polar ice!

Hot Stove Douglas

This was the name of a well-known Mayo miner. He was called "Hot Stove" because he had backed into a red-hot kitchen stove when he was drunk and had badly burned his buttocks.

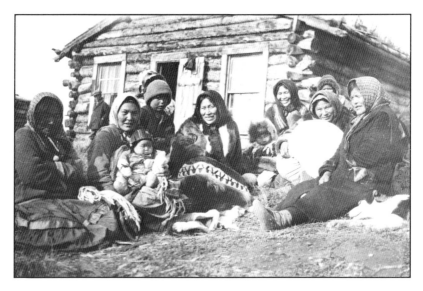

Some of my Indian patients

Fighting the Fuzzy Wuzzies

Officially, Shorty Carter was the hospital orderly and porter but in reality he was much more. He kept the boilers stoked with firewood; thawed frozen water pipes at sixty below; kept the vegetables in the root cellar from freezing; acted as policeman when the men got fresh with the nurses; and, invariably, got drunk Saturday nights. Shorty was born in East London and had short, very bowed, arthritic legs but he feared no-one. He told me that when he was young he fought the Fuzzy Wuzzies in the Sudan. He was too old to use guns but some of the patients said he was a wizard with a knife.

The man who loved cats

Joe Langtin was the Mayo water man. Every morning he filled his home-made wooden tank with fresh water drawn from a spring-filled well in front of my cabin and sold it to anyone who had no water—including me. For some reason his well never froze even when most of the other ones did. Joe was French-Canadian and if he was annoyed would speak French, rather than English. His horse, Elie, always got French and Joe's "marchez" could be easily heard half a block away. Elie was old, sway-backed and stubborn and so Joe would ask him, "Who gets your oats, eh?"— and Elie would start moving. We all loved Joe. The children would run out to feed Elie candy and went to visit Joe in his neat cabin, which was alive with cats.

Jack Dempster - Mountie explorer

Inspector Jack Dempster used to come to Mayo from Dawson for yearly inspections of the RCMP detachment. He was famous for his other annual inspection trips—from Dawson to the mouth of the Peel River at Fort McPherson, close to the Arctic ocean. These 400-mile journeys were made in winter with dog teams and

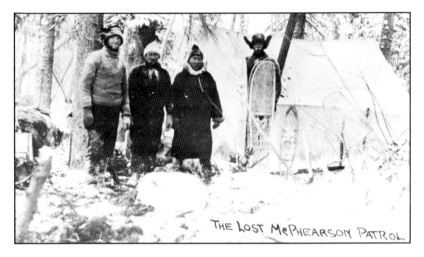

THE LOST McPHEARSON PATROL

The ill-fated Fitzgerald patrol

on one of them, in 1911, he found the bodies of RCMP Inspector
Francis Fitzgerald and his three men who got lost on the annual
mail patrol from Herschel Island to Dawson. The road from
Dawson to Inuvik was named the Dempster Highway in recogni-
tion of his skill and courage. Dempster was a quiet man who
smoked large, hand-made cigarettes. He stuffed so much tobacco
in them that his tunic was often sprinkled with tobacco. On one of
his trips he warned me that our friendship would never stop him
from discharging his duties. I could not understand what he meant
until I found out that he had heard that a group of us had been
shooting ducks and geese in the spring. The season, set by
international agreement, was in the fall, long after all the birds had
flown south. His warning had no effect.

Is it Constable, Cpl. or Sgt.?

The miners in Keno were a very tough bunch. They could hold
pneumatic drills in their hands for a whole shift or whack a steel
drill all day with a sledge-hammer, then get drunk, fight, and go

back to work next morning as if nothing had happened. Keeping these men in order was the responsibility of Constable, Corporal or Sergeant Ted McAskill. McAskill came from the New Brunswick McAskills, a family reputed to be able to outpull horses or lift platforms loaded with ten men. McAskill had a neck so muscled that it sloped from his huge shoulders right up to the base of his skull.

His only challenger was his friend Hard-Rock McDonald and if the two happened to be in a bar at the same time a fight was inevitable. After a few drinks, one would sniff the air and announce that he smelt a Dogan. The other would say something about a bloody Protestant. At this stage wise drinkers started to move chairs and tables to a discreet distance. Then McDonald would say that if McAskill was not in uniform he would wipe the floor with him. McAskill would take off his tunic and the fight would begin. After the loss of a tooth or two the two men would make up and spend the rest of the evening drinking together.

Headquarters in Dawson would hear about the fight and demote McAskill. But, since nobody could handle the miners like McAskill, he soon had his stripes back again.

A few graves to spare

Our Mayo mortician was, like his coffins, rough-hewn. Alex L'Esperance was essentially an entrepreneurial carpenter. He "undertook" to provide a grave and coffin, at a fee, for every funeral in Mayo. Like the rest of the country, the Mayo cemetery was situated on permafrost—darn hard grave-digging at any time of the year, and almost impossible at sixty below zero. The cemetery was divided into four sections, one each for Catholics, Protestants, Masons and Indians and each summer L'Esperance had to decide how many graves to dig in each section before fall freeze-up, for no Mason could be buried near a Catholic and no Catholic near a Protestant. The whole town watched the number and positioning of L'Esperance's graves. Let's see now, their thoughts ran, those three Catholic holes would have to be for Jones, Smith and O'Reilly and the two Masonic holes were for those old guys at Keno who had been looking bad all summer. But some years the guesses were wrong and L'Esperance had a few "dry holes" when summer came, graves destined to fill with water and become red ink items in L'Esperance's account book.

Bear hunter supreme

George Ortell, the man who showed me how to light a fire in the bush, didn't talk much but when he did he spoke about grizzly bears. To start with, he found them a good source of meat when cariboo and moose were scarce. Shooting them was simple in the winter. He'd find a hibernating bear by looking for the hoar-frost over its den and the dormant bear could be shot before it woke up. Ortell filled me in on a few details of their lives. As the weather gets colder food for the bears gets scarce. The combination of falling temperatures and less food, said Ortell, prompts them to find a cave or shelter under logs where they go to sleep. Very slow respiration and a very slow heart beat cause complete unconsciousness. Some of them, he said, can be rolled over easily. A few of the biggest and toughest grizzlies, however, seem to find some food in the late fall and do not hibernate. Their tempers worsen with the falling thermometer and so, Ortell warned, it is best to beware of a grizzly prowling about in January or February.

There is nothing that frightens Indians and trappers as much as grizzly bear prints in the winter snow. Ortell told me about a trapper whose foot was amputated and who strapped a grizzly's paw onto his stump. No-one ever went near his traplines!

PART TWO

WHITEHORSE

My empire—the hospital

The plane that brought me to Whitehorse landed on an icy
runway in the fading light of an early spring day. It was March,
1935, and I had left Mayo to become superintendent of the
Whitehorse hospital and the town's doctor. Any feelings of
importance vanished as soon as I stepped off the plane for there
was no-one from the hospital to meet me. I went to the Whitehorse Inn where the clerk put me in a room directly behind the
reception desk. He wanted me there, he said, "so I can get you by
knocking on the wall." Another inconvenience was the position
of the women's lavatory—just across the corridor from my door.
Many female patrons of the hotel's beer parlor turned left instead
of right as they hurried to answer nature's call and pushed into
my room in various stages of undress. I quickly put a sign on my
door pointing to the right door.

Soon after I arrived I had to meet the hospital board. The
chairman was Larry Higgins who was also the town's official
liquor vendor, a job which meant that he met almost everyone.

43

He briefed me on my duties which, simply stated, were to run the hospital on instructions from the board. Then there was Charlie Atherton, a pink-faced, balding Scotsman who worked in the grocery department of Taylor and Drury Stores. He was a middle-aged bachelor with a strong sense of duty, blue eyes and a complexion like a baby's bottom. Jack McPherson, the druggist, was also on the board. A jovial man, usually wearing a tam o' shanter, he was in charge of the hospital pharmacy and ordered many of the hospital supplies through his store. A few months later I asked the board why we had to get our supplies from him. Why not wholesale? Immediately I had an enemy on the board, with allies, for this would cut out the other merchants who sold supplies to the hospital. Frank Patterson, the bank manager, was another board member. He watched the costs. "Why," he asked one day, "had the consumption of toilet paper gone up?" I explained that several epidemics of dysentery had caused the increase in consumption.

Humour smells sweet

Soon after I arrived Larry Higgins gave me my first tough directive. He pointed out that every spring the hospital septic tank had to be cleaned out. What was I going to do about it? I told him that I would call the man who did it last year. Then Lauder Tully, the hospital porter, and Florence McDonald, the head nurse, told me that he had died; that was why the order had come to me. I tried all over town but nobody wanted to go down a ladder into a septic tank as big as a house. By this time I was up to my neck in work for, as in Mayo, I was the only doctor in town. Then I got another directive from the board. People living near the hospital were complaining about the smell. The board was challenging me and I was darn mad. So I sent out invitations to all the members of the board to be my guest at a grand septic tank cleaning on Saturday, May 6th at two o'clock. I would lead them

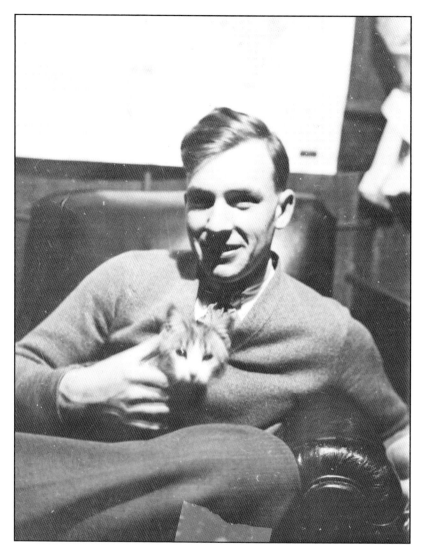

The author and Bugs the cat

down the ladder with the suction hose and each member of the board would have appropriate duties in sludge disposal. P.S. The wives of board members would be asked to provide light refreshments.

That did it. The whole town laughed and a man offered to do the job—and that is how I won my first battle with my new employers.

Whitehorse etiquette

After a few months the board rented a small house for me so that I could leave the noisy hotel. But the house had no insulation and only an old decrepit furnace. It was so cold that water froze in the house at night. There was no running water for houses in Whitehorse in the Thirties and the nurses at the hospital allowed me to use their bathroom provided that I agreed to wash off the ring after each bath. And I equipped my outhouse with a seat lined with rabbit fur that I had brought from Mayo.

With such a cold house I accepted any invitation to go out in the evenings but I found that the town's matrons did not like single men for two reasons: they were too cowardly to get married and support a wife (that meant an awkward number at the dinner table) and, of course, they could not be trusted with nubile daughters. I found out, too, that social life in Whitehorse was highly organized with a distinct pecking order. Mrs. J. McPherson, the druggist's wife, and her sister, Mrs. W. McBride, wife of the White Pass agent, were at the top of the pyramid and they gave dinners that were elegant for Whitehorse: fish courses with white wine; entrees with red wine; candles and crystal goblets on the table.

It took me a long time to get accepted but then Mrs. McPherson, who lived across the street, found out that I could play bridge. To make up even tables an "extra" was often necessary. "Doctor, could you drop in after the liqueurs?" would be my invitation to play bridge. Arriving about eight, I would find seven or eleven men and women obviously over-fed and sleepy, ready to start playing bridge. I would be ushered to the spare chair. This spare bridge player deal spread to other homes until one day I told Mrs. McPherson that if she wished me for bridge she had to feed me first. "Dear me, doctor," she protested. "We cannot have you to dinner. You have no partner." Quickly, I reassured her that my gastro-intestinal tract had no connection with my genito-urinary tract but I would be happy to eat by myself in either the dining room or kitchen. She agreed and from then on the matrons filled both the bridge chairs and my stomach.

Carcross cold shoulder

The town, isolated, with few diversions, was an unpleasant spot for a single doctor. Personality clashes were inevitable. The harder I tried the more unpopular I became. I realised that this was not my fault for I was constantly regaled with stories about the stupidity and indifference of the doctors before me. Sometimes I got into hot water for making decisions that I did not think were controversial at all. One of these involved a minor train accident at Carcross, about 40 miles to the south. After I had tended the injured men in the hospital I told the nurses that they did not have serious injuries and could go back to Carcross in a few days. There was an uproar. Nearly everyone in town thought I had been unfair and that I should have allowed the men to stay in the warmth and comfort of the hospital for some weeks.

One of my duties was to make regular visits to Carcross. I usually travelled by train and went first to the Indian residential school. The superintendent used to pick me up at the station, something I appreciated, for the school was a half mile or so up a dusty, sandy road. But on my first trip after the railway accident nobody came to meet me and I had to walk to the school, carrying my heavy black bag. The superintendent told me he would not help anybody who kicked out the railroad workers and from now on I could damn well walk back and forth to the train.

I spent that day, as usual, tending the sick children. When lunch hour came there was no food for me. On my way home, walking down the dusty road, I remembered the septic tank incident and realised that there was no way to complain without seeming petulant.

A few months later, however, I got a letter from the Indian Department, one of my many employers, telling me that the Carcross visits were entirely up to me. From then on I only went to Carcross if there was an emergency.

The dog it was that died

I was soon involved in another controversy that showed how difficult it was to please the good folk of Whitehorse. Late one evening I was asked to go up the railroad track a short way to see a boy who "had the colic." When I got to the cabin near the tracks I saw that my patient, Dennis Blaker, six or seven years old, was very ill. His distended belly pushed up the bedclothes and beside his head was a basin filled with faecal vomitus. His mother, who spoke with a strong English accent, said that he had complained of a belly-ache for several days. The pain had begun high in the centre of his abdomen and then moved down to the right side. It was obvious that he had a ruptured appendix–and probably general peritonitis.

I telephoned the hospital to get ready for surgery. Florence McDonald had just got back from skiing and she and the other nurse, Janet McTavish, helped Lauder Tully prepare the operating theatre. Jessie Howatt would come from her home to pour the ether. As I drove the boy to hospital I realised that he was probably going to die; without surgery he would certainly die; with surgery to remove his appendix he had a chance. But if I operated and he died I would probably have to leave Whitehorse. Resolution of the problem was easy: I had been taught that the doctor's first task is to save life and to ignore the consequences.

It seems trite to mention this rule but it has often stopped me wasting hours trying to make up my mind what to do.

We followed a strict routine at the hospital. Mrs. Howatt boiled the instruments in a copper clothes-boiler and checked the drapes and surgical gowns that had been boiled in bundles and dried in the hospital kitchen's oven. Then she helped us get the patient onto the operating table and started the anaesthesia. She was an expert in pouring ether and knew just how much to pour on the mask to avoid choking and still get the patient asleep. This usually took about half an hour and gave the surgeon and assistant nurse time to scrub up and put on their sterile gowns. At the right time Mrs. Howatt would say, "You may proceed now, doctor." I always gave the patient's skin a tweak to see if the anaesthesia was complete before starting surgery.

The operation to remove Dennis's appendix was routine. The rotting organ was cut out, the stump tied off and drainage tubes inserted to let the infection out. Despite my fears he started to get better and, after a month's convalescence during which he became the pet of the hospital, he returned home. I believe Dennis survived because of three factors: we had a good supply of intravenous fluids; his appendix was just under the belly wall and so only a short incision was needed; and the foul-smelling infection was caused by bacillus coli, of low virulence, and not by streptococcus.

My stock in the community went up when Dennis survived but a few weeks later it tumbled down again. Again the Blaker family was involved. They had a large malamute dog which had attacked a porcupine and got his mouth, face and throat full of quills. I was told the dog was good-tempered and so tried to pull one of the quills with pliers. He bit my hand. We tied the dog up between two trees and put him to sleep with ether. As I was taking out the quills in his pharynx I noticed that the poor dog was not breathing. He may have got too much ether or, more likely, the swelling caused by the quills in his throat had blocked his air passage. The Blakers did not forgive me—nor did the rest of the community. I may have saved a boy but I killed a dog.

TRANSPORT – YUKON STYLE

Danger in the air

When I had agreed back in Winnipeg to be a doctor in the Yukon I never realised how much the practice of medicine in the territory depended on transportation. Some patients had no means of getting to the hospital or doctor's office. In emergencies the only way to get the patient to hospital was by steamer or plane for there were virtually no roads and, anyway, the weather limited travel to certain months of the year. How to get the doctor and patient together, then, was a constant problem.

One bright summer morning the local telegraph operator sent me a message stating that some men had been injured when a plane had crashed near McDame, a small settlement on the Dease River to the southeast of Whitehorse. Everett Wasson, a local pilot, flew me there in a small Fairchild with pontoons. He had fitted the Fairchild with a high-power engine to lift it out of the water as quickly as possible—essential when working out of small lakes and narrow rivers. Wasson and I landed at McDame, tying up to a log boom in front of the Hudson's Bay store, and decided to walk to Trout Lake, the scene of the crash, to see the injured men and to check out the lake for a landing. Mosquitoes swarmed over us, biting any exposed surface and even going up our nostrils or into our mouths if we took a deep breath. Coming around a bend on a hillside we saw the tracks of a grizzly bear filling with ground water. Each paw-mark was so big that a man's hiking shoe could fit in it easily but what was worse was the sight of the water; that meant that the bear was very close indeed. We waited a while but the bear seemed to have gone and so we walked, very cautiously, to the crashed plane. It was a flying boat with a big single engine mounted above the centre of the hull.

The flying boat, loaded with a half dozen men, had tried to take off from Trout Lake, a reedy body of water that looked more like a swamp than anything else. It had cleared the water by twenty feet before crashing into some trees. One of the passengers had an injured shoulder and others had lacerated scalps with clotted blood all over their faces and hair. The pilot was in the worst shape. He had a concussion, certainly, possibly a skull fracture and was incoherent and difficult to manage. We tended to each of the injured: morphine for the worst and sedatives for the others. Then did some cleaning up and crude splinting.

Wasson walked back to McDame and flew the Fairchild to the lake and then began to ferry the injured, one at a time, back to McDame. The injured man was strapped in the seat beside Wasson and then he turned the plane so that it faced out into the lake. That done, we all held onto the tail of the plane while Wasson gunned the engine. When we could hold the bucking plane no longer we let go together. In what seemed an amazingly short time Wasson had the Fairchild on her "step," pulled back the stick with a jerk, settled a little back and took off just over the tree tops. He repeated this process until all of us were at McDame and we spent the night there in a Hudson's Bay shed.

The next problem was to get the lot of us back to Whitehorse. The Dease River in front of McDame is not very wide and it didn't have any long, straight stretches so Wasson selected the best spot and loaded half the passengers. Then he taxied downstream, faced the wind and opened the throttle. But the pilot of the crashed plane was delirious and would not stay in his seat. As he moved about he shifted the trim of the plane and made take-off impossible. So we had to strap him down. Wasson realised that he needed some controlled shifts in trim and told me to run forward and back in the plane at his signal. He hoped that shifting my weight at the right time would rock the plane onto the step of the pontoons. He was right. The plane shot forward when freed of the river's drag and we passed so close to the tree tops that I could see the cones on them. The engine was laboring so hard that I wondered if it could stand the strain of lifting us into the air. But it did. We flew on to Whitehorse and all of the crash survivors recovered.

Taxi service only

Wasson's plane was typical of the aircraft that we used to get around the Yukon. Nearly all of them were single-engined and switched from floats to skis to suit the weather. They were privately-owned, usually by their pilots, and provided a service similar to that of a taxi-service in a small town. The planes met the steamers to pick up and deliver goods and passengers and could be hired by anyone who needed to get somewhere quickly— and had the cash to pay for the trip. We hired a plane when there was an emergency and so did the various government departments or agencies like Indian Affairs or the RCMP. Some of the large mining firms had their own planes to transport bosses or urgently-needed supplies and we could use them. But we never knew when they might be coming or leaving and so they were of little value.

Soon after the outbreak of war the economy of the Yukon improved and the armed forces needed a better transportation system. As a result, small airlines were formed and regular services started. After a short while these small firms amalgamated or were taken over by Canadian Pacific Airlines and by the end of

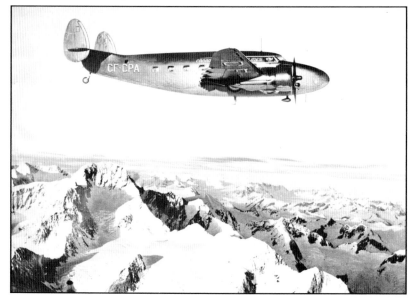

Over the mountains to Vancouver

the war there was regular service by twin-engined airliners between Whitehorse, Edmonton and Vancouver. Twice a week there was service to Dawson.

Sport on the stern-wheelers

Normally I and my patients had to use the river steamers. Six of them served three routes: Dawson to Whitehorse; Dawson to Fairbanks, Alaska; and Whitehorse to Mayo. They were stern-wheelers with boilers that burned four-foot spruce logs. These were cut the previous winter and stacked at intervals on the river bank. The stack had to be on the "cut bank" of the river (the vertical bank formed by current erosion) and about ten to fifteen feet above the water level, assuring a down-hill ride for the wood on the deck-hands' trolleys to the ship's deck. Watching the men go down the steep gang-plank with a huge load of wood was almost a sporting event. Speed was reduced by friction of the trolley's wheel against the boarded edge of the gang-plank. Then, with a sweeping curve, defying Newton's laws of motion, the load was dumped into a pit in front of the boiler. A little too much momentum, a missed turn, and the whole caboodle shot across the narrow bow into the river.

This load of fuel and the boilers were in the bow to balance the steamer's big reciprocating engines in the stern. Above the passenger accomodation midships was the wheel-house housing the pilot and captain and they communicated with the engineer down below in the stern by means of bells. One ring meant forward and two reverse. Speed was indicated by short jingles after the main signal. The steamer was steered by moving the main rudder under the stern as in other vessels. Our steamers, however, had a second set of rudders, called monkey-rudders, fixed behind and beneath the paddle wheel. They caught the slip-stream behind the wheel and were very effective in steering with minimum forward way. Piloting was a cinch when the steamer was laboriously pushing its way up-stream. Going downstream, when the stern-wheeler was pushed by the current, was much trickier and far more dangerous. A serious error could result in grounding or holing on a rock. A sunken steamer was rarely salvaged, for silt rapidly filled everything in the fast current, fixing the boat to the river bottom.

The stern-wheelers displaced only a few feet but they were constantly getting stuck on sand-bars. Experienced skippers used two tricks to get through shallow stretches of the river. One was to back over and let the paddle wheel dredge a channel through the sand-bar. This technique, however, usually bent or broke the monkey-rudders. The other trick was to use "crutches". These were two stout poles put into the water on each side of the bow.

Cables ran through pulleys on the tops of the poles to the bow steam winch and when the cables were tightened the bow was raised, allowing the vessel to squirm over the bar.

Shipboard sex = suffering

The officers on the steamers were old hands who returned to Whitehorse each spring like the ducks and geese. The deck-hands were usually young, healthy, university guys, often trying to make a buck to pay tuition fees.

Passengers were carried on all the steamers and many of them were women tourists. Put young men like these on board a small ship with female passengers and you had trouble for the doctor. Many of them, male and female, got gonorrhea. The first symptom they experienced was the feeling that they were urinating razor blades. I was always amazed by the behavior of the middle-aged female tourists in the Yukon spring. They had led sedate lives and then suddenly, in this new land, they would plunge into a torrid romance with a young fellow aboard a river steamer. Instead of asking his girl-friend to come and see his etchings, the deck-hand could ask her to come down to see the ship's engines. And, just aft of the engines, was a sick-bay ready for use with a couch and a door that locked.

Gonorrhea was also a problem among the older male passengers, the trappers and miners, who arrived on the steamers from Dawson. They suffered from urine retention and had to come to the hospital for catheterization. These men had had gonorrhoea and the infection, in pre-antibiotic days, could leave the tube permanently scarred, causing a stricture which had to be dilated repeatedly to prevent complete obstruction. We often used a rat-tailed catheter. The thin end of this two-foot tube usually passed even small strictures, safely guiding the progressively larger tube past the narrow stricture, until the "fat" end really stretched the scar. One man said the sensation was like having a baby through the penis!

Occasionally the Mounties asked me to see the bodies of men who had committed suicide and left notes saying they had done so because they could not urinate and were in agony. They let their dogs loose or shot them, locked their cabins, and blew their heads off. After seeing the first case, I insisted that every older trapper or prospector buy a medium-sized soft rubber catheter and carry it into the bush. When obstructed they simply lubricated the tube—usually with spit—and pushed it up the penis. The catheter was left in and when the bladder was empty the tube was knotted to prevent dribbling, then released as required. Some years later, when it was suggested the Yukon needed a new or revised coat of arms, I facetiously proposed that it should consist of two rampant catheters on a sea of fireweed.

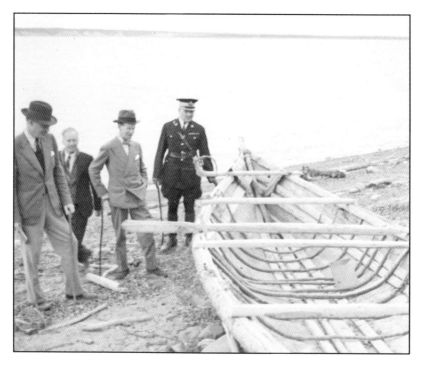

Visiting dignitaries inspect an Indian skin-boat

Pilot's tall tales

One of the steamer pilots, Kid Marion, was famous for his tall stories. Going down-stream the pilot house was off-limits to tourists. On the slower, up-stream trip they were allowed to go in and it was then that Marion recited his stories. One of them was about the way the river was eroding the bank and revealing the coffins and bodies of the men who had died in the rush to the gold-fields. Each spring, at places where the ship passed near a deep bank, Marion used to stick poles into the bank and then jam old boots on the poles so that they were flush with the earth. Marion, of course, knew the exact location of each "salted" bank. On the next trip at an appropriate place—a few miles from the "cemetery"—he would go into his spiel about the river and the coffins and corpses. Most tourists were sceptical and so Marion would slow the steamer as it passed the special bank. Then, casually, he would point to the protruding boots as proof of his story.

Everything came by ship

The stern-wheelers kept the whole of north-west Canada functioning in those days. They not only provided the best passenger transportation but also brought in nearly all of our food, clothes, equipment and last, but not least, booze. Meat was a real problem. It arrived in Whitehorse from Vancouver in frozen half-carcasses. It was refrozen in Whitehorse but was partially thawed when it reached Dawson and Mayo. Bacon was double-smoked down south to last a year but by spring bacon slabs that had been shipped the previous fall were heavily coated with pencillin mould. The locals got used to mould-covered bacon, just slightly rancid. Some said they even preferred it to the fresher kind. Eggs were shipped in a slimy solution called "water-glass." After a year they were slightly rotten but most people preferred them to the flat, fresh variety.

The first and last boats had special significance.

The first carried new supplies, fresh food and new faces, not to mention new flu bugs—and salesmen visiting the local stores for orders. The last boat, in contrast, was a sad occasion. It left Dawson in late September to churn its way up to Whitehorse in time to avoid getting stuck in the river ice. We said sad goodbyes to those going on holiday and really sad ones to friends leaving the north for good. On one such boat Inspector Jack Dempster and his family left the Yukon for good. Dempster had kept his lead dog—a very intelligent husky—as a house pet after he stopped going on his winter patrols and the dog was down at the wharf when the Dempsters left. The dog, which was cared for by another RCMP officer after Dempster had gone, never forgot that his master had left on a boat. For years it would stand on the dock howling at departing steamers, hoping, no doubt, to see Dempster again.

Last great run

In the late fall of 1937 the *Nisutlin*, a small, ancient stern-wheeler, was scheduled to make the last trip down river from Whitehorse to Dawson. At that time the Yukon Consolidated Gold Company was building a set of new gold dredges and needed lots of lumber before winter set in. The shipping firm decided to delay the *Nisutlin*'s trip until all the lumber was ready and then risk her in a dash down river just before the freeze-up. The old steamer was loaded to the water line with lumber and then her skipper literally tied down the throttle and sent off down the Yukon. Almost everyone in Dawson was watching for the *Nisutlin*, hoping she would not get frozen in and be wrecked when the ice broke up. She was sighted one September evening as she rounded the bend above Lousetown, the red light district. Exhaust steam mixed with sparks and small pieces of burning wood blew high above her stack as the old steamer smacked her way up to the dock, decks piled high with lumber. Crews worked all night unloading the lumber. Then the *Nisutlin* plowed her way through the slushy ice down to the shipyard and was pulled up the ways. She never sailed again. Next day the river was solid with shore to shore ice. Later some of the *Nisutlin*'s crew told how they had to stop the paddle-wheel at times to avoid hitting the herds of migrating caribou who were swimming the frigid river.

Sea-sick skipper

Another famous small steamer was the *Tutshi*, based at Carcross. Her master was Captain Tom McDonald and she plied the upper river lakes, carrying tourists up Lake Tagish to the head of the lake at Ben-Ma-Cree. Here there used to be a hotel run by the White Pass Company but it burned down and an old couple, the Partridges, were left there to serve refreshments— including their famous rhubarb wine—to Captain McDonald's tourists. All around their home were huge delphiniums and pansies that flourished in the rich alluvial silt under the continuous sunshine of the northern summer.

On one trip Captain McDonald, "Scotia Mac" to his friends, had on board a friend, a deep-sea captain named Palmer whose ship was tied up at Skagway. Palmer was taking an afternoon nap when the *Tutshi* ran into some choppy water at Windy Arm. Some of the passengers asked McDonald where Captain Palmer was. McDonald apologised for his friend and explained that he had become sea-sick and had to go below!

On another voyage a tourist asked Captain McDonald how they ran the *Tutshi* in the winter. He replied, "We simply drive spikes in the paddle-wheel boards to push her over the ice."

Second-class passengers use the rope

When the river systems were frozen Dawson was served by a weekly stage from Whitehorse. The stage consisted of a train of heavy sleighs pulled by a caterpillar-type tractor that followed a 400-mile trail along rivers, lakes and sloughs. Food and other supplies were kept from freezing by large buffalo furs and hot bricks. Passengers, covered with fur rugs, snuggled together on the sleighs. Those who couldn't afford to pay to ride on the sleigh could, for a few cents, use a rope attached to the last sleigh, tying the rope around their middle or just hanging on and walking. There were some medical prerequisites for travelling on the stage—with or without a rope. Constipation was a great help but bladder problems were a disqualification, for the tractor drivers liked to keep going, day and night. A toilet stop in the snow, with heavy clothes, was a terrible experience.

People taking the overland trip were always surprised to see water streaming out of some hillsides and over roads when the temperature was fifty or sixty below zero. As the water crossed the road it formed an impassable glacier. Roads to essential areas had to be kept free of glacier ice and it was done this way: an old diesel drum with a perforated bottom was placed at the spot where water came out of the hill. A small fire in the drum, tended regularly by road crews, warmed the water so that it ran over the road instead of on it.

Females preferred

The Indians, most trappers and some prospectors—and occasionally the Mounties—used dog-teams to get about. Sometimes I had to go with an RCMP dog-team to tend a sick man in the bush and learned a little about how the dogs work.

The dog next to the sleigh is called the wheel-dog and his job is to pull the sleigh to one side or the other to keep it in line with

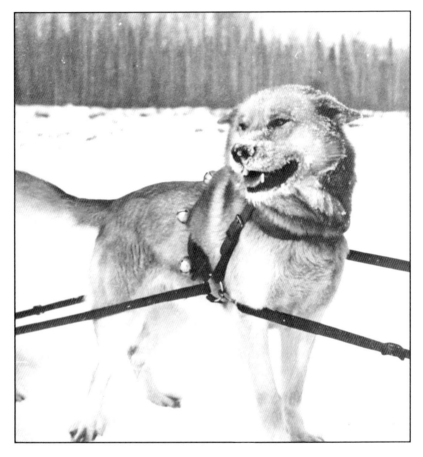

Yukon sleigh-dog: worker, not pet

the dogs ahead. He does this by moving his powerful rear end to keep the sleigh in line while running forward fast enough to prevent it from hitting him. The most important dog is the one in the lead—usually a female because females tend to be more intelligent and do not fight as much as the males. If you are crossing frozen lakes or rivers it's wise to watch the lead bitch very closely. If she starts whining, squirming or looking back it usually means that you are close to thin ice or ice bridging an air space above water.

I am sure that sleigh-dogs have a union. No. 1 in the rule book is a requirement that no member of a team shall urinate or defecate at the same time as any other member. When a team starts on a trip after a halt it goes about 100 yards and then one dog decides to attend nature's call. The rest of the team wait patiently until he or she is finished. Then, after a few hundred yards, another dog takes his turn until they are all comfortable. With six to eight dogs working together in this way the monotony of a trip can be broken a dozen times or so, with a few fringe benefits in the form of fights or sniffing sessions.

Our dogs were fed a frozen dried salmon a day and on this food could pull more than a hundred pounds each for several hours. The Indian sleighs were made of birch, sawed into slabs and held together with "babiche", the Achilles tendon of moose or cariboo. These threads were pulled through holes drilled obliquely through the boards so that they did not get rubbed through on the bottom of the sleigh. In the summer the Indians' dogs were converted into pack animals and I often saw them on the trail, trotting along with pots, pans and boxes tied on their backs.

The Yukon sleigh-dogs were bad-tempered and we never approached strange teams without a club in our hands. They were always given right of way on the trail. Occasionally the dogs seemed to have a sense of humour. One day I was travelling with an RCMP team when we were crossing a glacier. As we got to a patch of icy water the dogs suddenly swerved to avoid the water, tipping us off. Then the whole team made a U-turn on the solid ice, sat on their haunches and stared at us.

PART THREE

DAWSON

Marriage and a move

On August 17, 1936, the anniversary of the discovery of gold in the Klondike, Winona Spence and I were married in the little log church in Whitehorse. Winona was attended by her sister, Jean, from Winnipeg and my best man was Larry Higgins, the local government agent and liquor vendor. Larry was impatient to get the ceremony over so that he could get back to selling booze to a ship-load of tourists who had just arrived. The clergyman had the jitters. He was a young man who had recently taken over the Whitehorse parish and he confided to me he had buried both Indians and white men but never before married a white man. Two weeks later, after Winona had opened up the last of her barrels of dishes and wedding presents, Bruce Watson, the local telegraph operator, brought me a telegram.

"Well, Bruce," I said, "what does the harbinger of fate bring today?"

"Allan," he replied, "your life is about to round a sharp bend in the river. Dr. Nunn has died in Dawson and you're to be on a special plane for Dawson in a few hours."

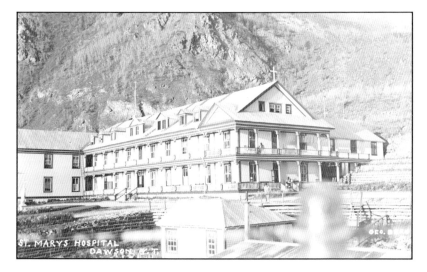

St. Mary's Hospital in Dawson

Dr. Herbert Nunn had been the only doctor in Dawson, responsible for the entire northern Yukon region, including the 900 men working on the Dawson dredges. Later I found that he had died of peritonitis from a ruptured appendix. There was no-one in Dawson who could operate on him in time and the delay had killed him.

A couple of hours later I got a telegram from Mr. G. Jeckell, Comptroller of the Yukon, telling me that Everett Wasson would fly me immediately to Dawson as a woman was in labour there. The doctor at Tulsequah, a village in the Stikine area, would replace me in Whitehorse. I had been given no chance to say whether I wanted to leave or not and had to leave Winona in a strange town, sharing the house with my Scotty, Angus, who would have nothing to do with her.

Snow was already covering the higher peaks as Wasson and I flew north. As I got out of the float-plane I was welcomed by Mr. Jeckell, Charlie McLeod and Warren McFarland, the two men who ran the large dredging company whose employees I would attend. I was rushed by car up to the big hospital on the hill to see a maternity case, Mrs. Evelyn Craig, about to have her second child, and after checking her condition I took a look around the hospital run by the Sisters of St. Anne. It was full of the gold company's men, patients from the town, with a ward for men and women in extended care.

The three men who met me on the dock, with Mr. L. Wernecke, manager of Treadwell Yukon Gold mines, ran the Yukon in those days. They had decided my fate, and, thank goodness, Winona went along with their decision. She repacked her barrels of dishes, muzzled the dog, and a week later set sail down the Yukon to Dawson to join me.

Class and indoor toilets

In 1936 Dawson was still the capital of the Yukon—politically, financially and socially. George Black from Dawson represented the Yukon in Ottawa and was Speaker of the Commons. Our major industry, gold dredging, was a prosperous business while the rest of the country suffered in the hungry Thirties. Socially, Dawson had a pecking order worthy of a large city.

Caesar wrote that Gaul could be divided into three parts but Dawson could be divided into two parts, those with running water in their homes and those without. The latter group found it difficult to climb socially while they had to carry this stigma. Any family who exposed their posteriors to the Arctic winds could not expect to reach the top echelons of Dawson society. Of course, we had other divisions. The town had a proud history going back to the gold rush when more than 15,000 people lived in Dawson City. This left us with a horde of government officials who perpetuated such traditions as designated "days at home," visiting cards and a rigidly-enforced pecking order.

The civil servants and politicians were at the top. This group included Comptroller Jeckell, Mr. and Mrs. George Black, the officer commanding the R.C.M.P. and other federal employees.

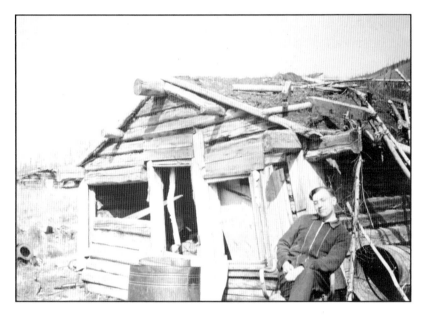

The author eyes a potential summer home

At the second level were the Bishop of the Anglican Church, the Bishop of the Catholic Church and Chief Justice McAuley. A little below these came the professionals: doctors, lawyers, engineers and bankers. The third group contained merchants and the members of similar professions. This group was large and much more fun, even if they could not pass the water test. Then, of course, there were the ordinary folk who did most of the work. The social stratification was rigid. If you were in doubt about your rank you could find out by noting the position allotted you in the Grand March at the New Year's Ball. Before the dancing began everybody marched in a great circle. In the lead came the King's representatives; then came the clergy, police and professionals, all solemnly shuffling forward, followed by the shopkeepers.

Another social custom was the "at home" convention. The senior matrons had commandeered a certain monthly date to be "at home." This was defined, not as a set date but as, say, the second Tuesday of each month. A woman visiting on "at home" days had to bring three cards, two with her husband's name neatly embossed on them and one with her own. All of the cards were dropped into a container that already held all the cards from previous visitors. I never found out what happened to them when the container was full! Dinner parties were first-class affairs and most hostesses insisted on tuxedos for the men and evening gowns for the women. Even a small party called for candles at the table and the china and silver was the best.

Fresh meat and greens

The big challenge for a hostess was to get fresh meat, fresh fruit or green vegetables such as lettuce or celery. These could be only obtained by bribing the pilots of the occasional bush plane that came to Dawson. My wife once wangled a few grapefruit from a Whitehorse friend who sent them by plane. She cut the grapefruit in half, freed each section and put a maraschino cherry in the centre. When I saw how smart they looked I had an idea. The day before I had noticed a box of beautiful glass eyes in a cupboard at the hospital. Allan Fraser, a friend, kept Winona out of the kitchen while I replaced the cherries with the glass eyes, buried in the grapefruit so just the glassy pupils showed. Fraser and I then served the guests with an extra round of doubles to prepare them for the shock. Eventually, in the dim candle light, we produced our grapefruit. The eyes looked real but no one was fooled enough to try and devour them.

To provide some variety in our menus most of the men tried to kill moose or cariboo. We could get lots of salmon for there were several runs up the Yukon River from the Bering Sea each year. The fish were caught in wheels anchored at bends in the river. A large salmon cost twenty-five cents in Dawson. Most of the fish was dried and stacked like firewood and used as dog food.

For fuel we bought spruce and birch; three-foot lengths for the furnace and small pieces for the kitchen stove. We had a few thieves who did not mind borrowing from someone else's wood pile. One miner solved this problem by drilling a marked fire-log and putting in a dynamite cap. The culprit was the fellow whose stove blew up. And there was a saying in Dawson that a gentleman was a man who cut his firewood in small pieces so that it could be easily handled by his wife.

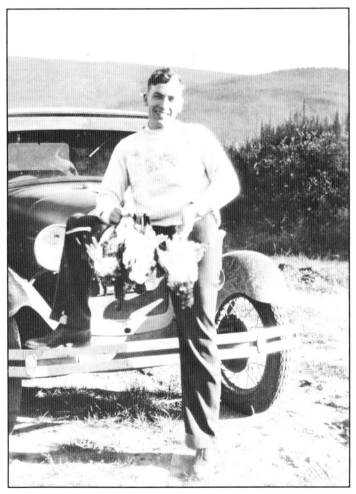

Hunter's bag—some white-ringed ptarmigan

MADAMS IN CHARGE

Sporting girls must be discreet

Everyone in Dawson used the same method of keeping an eye on their neighbours: they watched the chimneys. If no smoke could be seen you knew something might be wrong. One Christmas morning Winona and I and our three children were opening gifts when the telephone rang. A man from the north end of town had noticed the fire was out in a cabin belonging to a former prostitute. I didn't want to leave my warm home on Christmas Day but as the man sounded really worried I bundled myself up in heavy clothing and walked to the woman's cabin. The front door was unlocked and inside I found the woman lying partially covered on the bed, frozen to death. An empty whisky bottle sat on a table beside the bed; there was no fire, little furniture and no food. It was a pathetic ending for someone who, when she was young and beautiful, had been desired by so many men.

Prostitution was illegal in the Yukon but, with men out-numbering women roughly three to one, it wasn't surprising that the sporting girls, as we called them, were allowed to ply their trade as long as they did so discreetly. There were about 26 of these girls in Dawson, working in three houses managed by efficient, aggressive madams. Both the madams and the Mounties wanted to keep venereal disease in check and so I went on the RCMP payroll as Acting Assistant Surgeon. I inspected the girls regularly and acted as liaison officer between the madams and the law. A few days before holidays or long weekends the madams would send their girls to my office for inspection. The suspect ones were checked, smears taken and, if healthy, given a certificate. This document stated that at a certain date and hour the individual was deemed free from venereal disease and fit for duty. Most of the girls co-operated and came to my office for inspection and stopped work while they were being treated. For those who did not we had ways of enforcing their sexual isolation and preventing them from spreading disease. Legally, they could be charged under the Prostitution Act or a section of the Contagious Disease Act but neither of these was very effective. We had a much better weapon. If a girl refused to co-operate we black-listed her. A man coming into town on a spree often had to see the doctor for a medical problem and as he was leaving the office he was advised to avoid that particular girl. Then the number of her customers would start to fall, she would get the message and come to my office for treatment.

Everywhere - beads and dolls

If there was trouble in a brothel or someone was hurt the madam would phone my office. My job was to see that the injured were treated and that there was no unnecessary publicity. One cold evening I received a call to go to Ruby's brothel to see an injured man. I had another doctor, Dr. Geoff Homer, working with me for a short time and I asked him to come with me because I was told that the patient had injured his head and was bleeding badly. We knocked on the outer door and then stepped into a hallway from which two doors led to the brothel. Ruby inspected us through an aperture in the floor above, gave the signal and a pretty, dark-haired young woman let us into a large parlour stocked with the usual gaudy furniture and strings of beads. The beads gave the room a slinky atmosphere that was made worse by scores of dolls, usually with flaring skirts, perched on sofas, cupboards and tables.

Sitting in the centre of the parlour was a large, muscular man bleeding profusely from a scalp wound. The dark-haired girl told us, in a French accent, that he had fallen and hit his head on a bedside table. The wound was superficial and so Geoff asked the girl for a basin of warm water in English. As she did not appear to understand, we used our limited French to get the water and two other girls brought it in. We cleaned the man's wound and got ready to leave. But then the girls stopped chattering to each other and Geoff and I thought we heard sounds in the kitchen. The wound was still bleeding a little and this gave us an excuse to find out what was going on. We asked, "Plus d'eau chaude, s'il vous plait," and without waiting for the girls to reply went into the kitchen. Sitting around a table were half a dozen of the most prominent men in town. We went around the table shaking hands. "Good evening, Bill. Greetings, Jim. Welcome back to Dawson, Harry."

At that time I was being unjustly criticised by some of the older matrons in town. I knew that a few of my predecessors had been run out of town by petitions, gossip and innuendo coming from these women who had too much time on their hands. Now it was my turn to apply a little pressure. After fixing up the bleeding man we all had drinks in the kitchen and struck a deal: Geoff and I would keep our mouths shut and the men we caught in Ruby's place would curb their wives' tongues. Both sides kept their sides of the bargain.

I'll take it in trade

A friend came to my office one day and shyly explained that

he thought he had venereal disease. This surprised me, because he was the last man I suspected of cheating on his wife. He explained that when his regular work had run out he reached an agreement with Ruby to put storm windows on her brothel. All was well while he worked on the ground floor but when he started on the second floor he could watch the girls at work. He was so intrigued that when he finished his work he turned down the cash payment and told Ruby that he wanted time with the girls instead. Now he was paying for that decision. I told him to make excuses to his wife and after a few treatments his symptoms had gone.

Amateurs spoil business

The girls often complained about amateurs stealing business from them. They particularly resented the activities of a young Dawson woman who was, apparently, available to almost anyone. This woman told me she could not sublimate her sex drive in any way and could think about little except sex. I thought she just lacked will-power until one day she came to the office for a routine pelvic examination. I discovered a tumour about the size of a goose egg on one of her ovaries. Cancer was a possibility so I removed the tumour but the pathological reports showed the growth was actually producing a huge excess of female sex hormone. After the operation she started behaving very differently. The men around town were baffled. They couldn't understand why someone who had been such an easy conquest suddenly had become as cold as the Arctic winter.

Soldiers mean business

One day, soon after the United States entered the war, two steamers filled with American soldiers came to Dawson. As the stern-wheelers tied up at the dock the soldiers started shouting and cheering. Things were quiet in Dawson in those days and so most people in town, including my wife, sons and myself, went down to the dock for the show. The officer in charge was a dentist, I discovered, and was chiefly concerned with seeing that his men did not get too far away from the ship. They could disembark but not leave the dock area. A number of sporting girls saw their chance and took up positions in the bush on either side of the road from the dock. They were soon joined by some of the soldiers. After a while the officer saw his men disappearing into the bush and then coming back to the ship with smiles on their faces. "What the hell's going on?" he shouted so that we could all hear. When he was told he ordered the military police on the steamers to get the men back and send the girls packing. Then he came over to me and said he'd been told I was the town doctor. Some of his men had "escaped" and had been exposed to venereal disease. Would I examine them?

I went to the hospital and one man appeared. Since some of our sporting girls did have gonorrhea I gave him a prophylactic injection of argyrol, a black solution of a silver salt. As I was leaving I heard a man marching a group of soldiers into the entrance hall. He came in and said, "Sorry, Doc, but all these guys have been exposed and need treatment." Sister Faustina, who was helping me, boiled up some more catheters and prepared some more argyrol. As each man came into the room the sergeant gave him a tongue-lashing. "Imagine you, Smith, fornicating with some whore up in this country. You with a wife and kids at home, exposing yourself to the clap or worse." The last man was a tiny chap and the sergeant said to him, "And you, Jones. What are you doing getting mixed up with these chippies? How the hell could you handle these big women, anyway?"

Finally the last man was treated and sent back to the ship. The sergeant shut the door, turned to me, and said, "Guess you had better give me a shot, too, Doc."

Ruby's recovery room

I shouldn't give the impression that all my dealings with sporting girls were serious. They had their humorous moments too. Just after the war I spent a month doing some surgery in a Catholic hospital in Vancouver and Ruby came south for a minor operation. She was confused about hospital routine and asked me all kinds of questions. Most were easily answered but she insisted on knowing where she had been put during her recovery from the anaesthetic. She said she had awakened "drunk" in a big room filled with other "drunk" men and women. I explained that all people who were recovering from anaesthetics were put in one room, with special staff, until they were fit to go to their own rooms. We called it the recovery room. Ruby was well liked by the nursing sisters who never knew what she did in Dawson and before going home she gave a wheelchair to the hospital.

When I was back in Dawson I went to Ruby's brothel to see a sick woman. Ruby had just spruced up her house, painting the rooms and installing new furniture. On the second floor there was a landing from which corridors led to the bedrooms. This landing had been made particularly luxurious with new settees, table lamps and the inevitable dolls. I complimented Ruby on the decor and asked why she had lavished so much effort on the landing. "Monsieur le docteur," she said, smiling, "this is our recovery room!"

Then there was the time a premier from Eastern Canada visited Dawson. We were told that he would be accompanied by members of his Cabinet and top civil servants and so a big reception was planned to which everyone who mattered was invited. The chartered plane arrived but none of the dignitaries managed to find their way to the reception. We all waited for an hour then ate the sandwiches and crooked our little fingers as we drank our tea with no-one special to see us. I went back to the hospital to work and later, in need of a rest, went to Gleaves' cafe for a sandwich and cup of coffee. One of the sporting girls was there, also in need of a rest and a bite to eat. She told me that she and her fellow-workers had been busy servicing the plane-load of important visitors and, in her opinion, they were in no shape to go anywhere or meet anyone until the morning.

FIGHTING EPIDEMICS

Watching the water

I also had to battle another potential health hazard—Dawson's water supply. The pumping station was a large building in south Dawson, directly across the Klondyke River from Lousetown. Water from a well sunk in the station floor was pumped through the mains. The well was separated from the Klondyke River by a gravel and sand barrier that seemed to give adequate filtration. However, the well often proved inadequate, especially when everybody had their overflows operating in winter to keep pipes from freezing. Then water was pumped directly from the river into the mains. Three huge dredges worked up-river from Dawson busily digging up gold-bearing gravels. The gold was washed out and the waste gravel (called tailings) was dumped in rows from the stern of the dredge's hull. Unfortunately more than gravel was being returned to the Klondyke, for each dredge had a convenient outhouse suspended over the dredge's stern. When I saw that the nearest dredge was operating only a short distance from the city's pump-house I realised that when the level of water was low in the well, raw sewage was being pumped into the city mains.

80

I wrote a letter to Comptroller Jeckell, with a copy to the manager of the Dawson Utilities, pointing out the danger of an epidemic from contaminated drinking water. They replied that this had been going on for years and that nobody had worried before. Well, I was worried, for the neck to be stretched, if typhoid broke out, was mine. I could not resign as medical officer of health, for there was no other doctor to take the job. Devious methods had to be used. My wife began to boil our drinking water and we made sure that our neighbours knew. If anyone asked we made no accusations; we just kept boiling the water, making everyone curious.

Then a stranger arrived in town and started to snoop around the waterworks and to take water samples. Nobody paid attention to him until he insisted on drinking only bottled or boiled water. What's more, the hotel staff reported, he brushed his teeth only in purified water and even put a chemical in his bath water. Soon everybody discovered that the stranger was an engineer from Ottawa. His personal precautions showed that he was going to condemn the water supply. I never saw his report but a week after he left Dawson work started on a new well.

Army battles typhoid

As I was the only doctor in the northern Yukon I had to perform the duties of a medical officer of health. That meant I had to keep an eye on everything from garbage disposal to infectious and contagious diseases. I was scared that the region would be exposed to an epidemic of typhoid, diptheria, polio or some other communicable disease. How could one man handle an epidemic and, at the same time, do surgery, maternity and other medical work?

We had an epidemic of polio in 1944 but there was only one case of paralysis. The worst problem was fear. The next scare concerned typhoid fever. At the time Whitehorse was overflowing with thousands of American soldiers and airmen en route to Alaska and the Aleutians. Some Soviet airmen were also there picking up planes to fly to Siberia. Dawson, on the other hand, was a quiet little place hundreds of miles away. One morning when I visited the hospital Sister Faustina told me she had admitted a young Indian girl who had come across the Mackenzie mountains from Aklavik. She seemed to have typhoid fever. I sent off a stool specimen to Vancouver with instructions to check for typhoid bacilli. The laboratory report was positive and it was intercepted by the U.S. army medical corps in Whitehorse. A horde of Army doctors arrived in Dawson at the same time as the report was delivered. They demanded that the whole community be vaccinated at once. That made sense and I agreed. The Eagle Community Hall was cleaned up and typhoid vaccine flown in along with syringes and needles. I had to shoot a cubic centimetre of the murky fluid into hundreds of arms. Several women said they did not want their shot in the arm. This produced a routine reply from the military policemen who were supervising the mass vaccination: "O.K., madam. Then pull up your dress and take it in the rear." The arms had it! Happily, there were no more cases of typhoid.

MOUNTIES' MAN

Military style

My salary for being the RCMP's Acting Assistant Surgeon was small but the duties were substantial. Basically I had to do anything they wanted me to do—attend court cases, assist in investigations, answer complaints and look after sick personnel.

The Mounties followed a military pattern, with lots of spit and polish, reports to write, and strict inspections. Every Saturday morning while I was in Dawson the contingent—an assistant commissioner, some officers and about 24 constables—went on parade and I had to be there. Part of the ceremony consisted of raising the flag. There was a small cannon at the foot of the flag staff and I was just bursting to have somebody important visit us so that we could shoot it off. No luck; it remained silent through the years. Then we all inspected the jail where most of the prisoners were on drunk and disorderly charges. The next stop was the mess. We all trailed from the lock-up into Johnny Dine's neat kitchen and from there to the sleeping quarters. Each bed was neatly made up with the man's private box at the foot. The constable stood at attention in full uniform while we peered at him as we passed by. Periodically, the officer commanding gave the men a little talk after he or his wife had heard through the grapevine that one of his boys had been "keeping company" with an ineligible woman—someone's wife or a sporting girl. It went something like this: "Discretion is to be your guide in your relations with the town women. If you are indiscreet and the force hears about it, out you go on the next boat."

My closest association with the RCMP came during our yearly tour from the Arctic coast down to the Alaskan panhandle and the Liard River and one of my unofficial tasks was to warn the men by radio that their boss was on his way. This gave the lone constable or corporal time to get his papers in order, find his red-serge uniform, brush off his Stetson hat and get shaved. Many of the men in the bush never shaved for months. Whiskers helped to break the winter wind and kept off the voracious mosquitoes. At each post we visited the Mountie or Mounties were waiting at the small pier to catch the tethering rope from the plane and salute their commanding officer. Each man looked funny with tanned skin on his forehead, nose and around the eyes contrasting with the pure white rest of his face—the result of the emergency shave! It was traditional for officers to ignore this evidence of a beard but if the barracks, jail or office was not neat, there was hell to pay.

Blind and crippled

While the officer heard minor court charges in his capacity as magistrate, my job was to see the sick, mostly Indians. There were always teeth to pull, so the dental syringe and forceps were kept at the ready. On a trip to Carmacks one year the local Indian Chief asked me to see a blind Indian girl. She was in a tent by herself on the outskirts of the camp. The girl was brought to us draped across a saddled horse; head, arms and chest on one side, the rest of her body hanging over the saddle on the other side.

When her family lifted her off the horse, I realised that her hip joints were fused solid at a right angle to her body by tuberculous bone disease. When she was put on the ground she shuffled ahead, bent forward like a four-legged animal, her gloved hands feeling her way at ground level. All this and totally blind. Buck Stone, the pilot, who had come with me, turned pale and vomited.

I examined her. The damage caused by TB to her hips and eyes was all too obvious. There was nothing to be done except take care of her, but where? Back in Dawson, I wrote to Ottawa complaining about the lack of any facilities to help the girl and many others like her. Tongue in cheek, I suggested euthanasia. Officials in Ottawa replied that there was no place for her and rejected, deadpan, my suggestion of euthanasia. Later, thanks mainly to church groups, help was obtained in local hospitals and at Edmonton for this poor girl and other Indians like her. Then the discovery of streptomycin and other drugs just after the war almost entirely eliminated the dreadful suffering that TB could cause.

God help this old woman!

The young blind girl accepted the little aid we offered her but on another trip I met an old blind woman who refused to let us help her. We had landed at Aishihik Lake, near Whitehorse, where the Indian band had nearly starved the previous winter. A few months later a mysterious epidemic had killed off most of the younger members of the band. The buildings were deserted. Not even a dog could be seen. The only sign of life was a flock of adult swans with cygnets nesting in a small arm of the lake. As we checked the cabins we found a frightened old Indian woman. She was totally blind and was squatting near a small fire that heated an old lard pail containing water and what appeared to be gopher or squirrel. Sheets of dried meat were hanging from a tree but her small tent contained no food, only a few old blankets. Attached to the entrance flap of the tent was a note reading, "This old woman too sick to travel; we must go; God help this old woman; God help you." It was signed, "Sam Williams." We tried to get her to leave with us on the plane but she would not go. We left her food and I gave her a large pack of matches which we could see made her

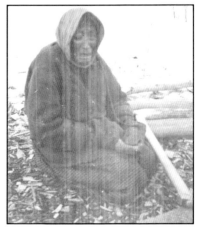

Blind old woman left to die

happy. Then we took off, sadly realising that she would probably freeze or starve to death. God may have helped this poor old woman. We certainly did not.

Starving, yet hospitable

One summer our annual tour included Snag on the White River, a community that got its name because of its heavy burden of silt. Snag also had the dubious reputation of being the coldest spot in North America. Our plane pulled up near a neat log cabin from which a Swedish man came out to greet us. He was painfully thin and looked ill. The police interrogated him about a missing man. When the questioning was over, the man invited us to join him for supper. We began with a drink of Aquavit and then he opened a can of his precious butter to put on the hard biscuits and fried grayling that formed the main course. For dessert we had stewed rhubarb. This man, a prospector, had poled these supplies up the miserable, silt-ridden White River to his cabin. He was obviously nearly starving, yet when several over-fed men from Dawson came along, he didn't hesitate to bring out his precious food supply. This was Yukon hospitality.

On the way back to Dawson, we decided to send in groceries and fresh produce to him, as the plane was returning to Snag the next day.

Lum gets a cure

Another inspection tour to Snag yielded an unusual case involving an Indian boy, Lum, who we had been told, had "matter running out of his head." Lum was about five and would not let us get near him, so he was caught and brought out of the bush. The owner of the Snag trading post had been keeping this child for years hoping to obtain medical help for him. Lum had earache and large amounts of matter oozed from the ear canal as well as from several holes in the scalp behind his ear. We could do nothing for him in Snag and so persuaded him to let us take him to the Dawson hospital along with the storekeeper who had befriended him. The boy was terrified. The nurses and sisters cleaned him up and got him into bed and for a week we just applied clean dressings and tried to develop his confidence.

X-rays showed that a large piece of dead tubercular bone was the source of Lum's trouble. For the next few months the sisters and nurses got Lum well, physically and mentally. He picked up some English, helped about the hospital and became everyone's favorite. Finally he was strong enough for an operation. I decided to cut the scalp in a wide crescent behind the ear and then pull the ear forward. Very gently I grasped the dead piece of bone and was relieved to find that it was quite loose. As I tried to free it a sharp splinter of bone appeared. This could easily pierce the dura (the outer membrane covering the brain) which I could see pulsating in the hole. If I simply pulled out the decayed bone with its splinters I could easily cause a fatal haemorrhage so I steadily clipped away at the edges of the bone until it dropped out, with Lum's middle-ear bones attached. I stitched up the wound loosely, leaving a soft spot in the skull.

Lum recovered and was renamed Jim. The last time I saw him he was happily playing with other children in a Dawson schoolyard. As I watched I prayed that nobody ever hit that soft skin behind his ear.

Brave little girl

A few days after finding Lum we stopped at Francis Lake where I was soon hard at work extracting teeth. This wasn't an easy job, especially as the Indian women, accustomed to chewing their husbands' mukluks to soften them after they had dried hard, had worn the crowns of their teeth level with the gums.

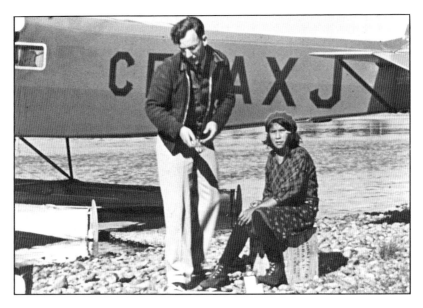

Pulling teeth on RCMP patrol

When I had finished, a shy girl about ten years old showed me her hand. Her palm was grossly distended with her fingers, also swollen, sticking out like prongs. She said she had fallen against a tree and impaled her hand on a protruding branch. A piece of wood was buried in her palm and her friends could not pull it out.

How to get the wood out and drain the palm? I carried syringes with cartridges of Novocaine for dental extractions but local anaesthetic is not very effective in such infections and so I just used it to "freeze" the skin. After considerable exploring, I removed a piece of wood about an inch and a half long and a half inch wide. This brave little girl never whimpered, despite the fact that the only anaesthetic was a small amount of Novocaine in the swollen skin. Some years later, I saw the girl in Dawson. Her hand had healed well but her fingers were a little stiff.

The death of Jim Croteau

Jim Croteau shouldn't have died the way he did. He was a trapper, placer miner and professional hunter, a tall, lean man with a walrus moustache who didn't talk very much. In the fall of 1939 he was killed in a gun battle with the Mounties near his cabin at Jensen Creek.

The Dawson RCMP had asked me to go with them because they thought there'd be some bloodshed. They were right. On the way Assistant Commissioner Sandys-Wunch explained that Croteau had been quarreling with mail carrier George Fulton over deliveries. When Croteau threatened to shoot Fulton the next time he came down the road, the police were called in. As Croteau was a deadly shot with a rifle at any distance the police went to Jensen Creek in full force, rifles at the ready. Croteau shouted from his cabin that he would shoot anyone who approached the place. When the Mounties started to close in, Croteau suddenly bolted from the building, firing a round into the air for emphasis.

Croteau took cover near a hunting shelter he had built close to a moose-lick and began firing in the direction of the police. I couldn't believe he was trying to kill anyone for he was too good a shot to keep missing. Suddenly, all hell broke loose. The police were firing round after round and Croteau was trying to keep

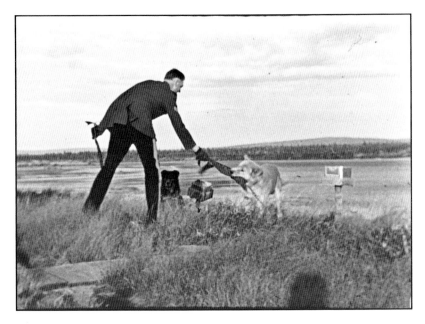

RCMP Sgt. W. Bayne feeds sleigh-dog at Old Crow

pace with them. I was lying at the bottom of a deep ditch and hugged the ground so hard that gravel got inside my shirt. A bullet nicked Sandys-Wunch's ear. He became furious and his next shot hit Croteau's leg, almost taking his knee off. But Croteau got madder and kept on firing. Then a bullet struck Croteau's chest, fatally wounding him.

We found Croteau's body slumped behind a log. His death seemed so unnecessary. I was certain that if someone had quietly spoken to Croteau in his cabin the whole quarrel could have been resolved.

Prayer for a boy

Late one fall a trapper named Anderson arrived in Dawson by river from Forty Mile, an abandoned gold mining settlement at the mouth of the Forty Mile River, about twenty miles down-river from Dawson. He had come to tell the RCMP that he had found the body of a young man washed up on a sand bar near his cabin. Corporal Ken Bond and I were told to go to Forty Mile to investigate. We went in Anderson's elongated river canoe, not much more than a hollowed-out log with a small outboard motor at the stern. Black scurrying clouds obscured the sun with only an occasional patch of light filtering through. The wind whipped up waves about a foot high that splashed against the narrow, low boat and the spray immediately froze on our clothes, weighing the canoe down even more. Whirling in the dim light above us, migrating cranes made their way south. They flew in a wide circle, looking like a tornado as they gradually moved southward. It was too windy and stormy for ducks to be flying but high in the sky the majestic, more organized geese were also flying south.

At last we reached the boy's body. I could find no signs of violence but he was wearing rubber hip-waders, a disastrous mistake. When he was dumped from his boat in the Forty Mile rapids the legs of the waders would have filled with water and even the best of swimmers would have drowned. The ground was frozen solid so we could not bury him there. Lower down the sandy river bank, however, was a strip of soil that would do us fine. The three of us soon dug a grave. We put the body on a sheet of old corrugated iron roofing and lowered him into the grave. With a last look at this handsome, young man—just a boy—we placed a blanket over his body.

There was an awkward moment when not one of us wished to start covering the body. Bond looked up and said to me, "Say something." I thought how transient and uncertain our existence on this earth really is and how helpless we are to change things. There had to be some way of showing our feelings for the loss of this boy and if the expression was to mean anything it had to reflect our beliefs about after-life. After a few moments I turned to Bond and said, "Let's just say the Lord's Prayer." A long time before, at the University of Manitoba, I had to put the Lord's

Prayer into Latin as part of an examination. Some sentences were easy, but that part about not doing the things we ought to have done and doing the things we ought not to have done was a real corker for gerunds and subjunctive tenses. No wonder I remembered it! We mumbled through the prayer and, with the sleety wind in our faces, filled in the grave. Then we marked the spot with a crude cross.

The trip back to Dawson was dangerous. Anderson's small boat had to fight an icy current churned by a head wind and we were covered with freezing spray. The next morning the Yukon was solid with ice and it remained that way for eight months. Even the geese and cranes were gone, leaving the land to the silence of the Arctic winter.

Secret of the skulls

Early one fall, when the cariboo were running, I went out with friends to hunt for winter meat. We parked the truck near the Alaskan border and each man took his rifle and set out in search of the cariboo. I walked several miles along a ridge. Only a few stunted spruce trees had survived the vicious winds of winter but the ground was not barren for it had an attractive covering of red squaw-berries growing out from a mass of dark green leaves that waved in the wind. Flocks of ptarmigan were feeding on the berries. They were already changing to their white winter feathers. The thin bright red flash above their eyes, however, was not changing. I often wondered what this red streak was designed to do. Was it a sort of light-absorbing patch like football players use to protect their eyes from glare? Or was it a beauty mark like the mascara women use?

I enjoyed being alone on these wind-swept ridges, realizing my own insignificance. And then, while I was walking along a ditch-like depression, I looked up and saw two bleached human skulls. One was of an adult; the other of a half-grown boy or girl.

The rest of the skeletons were partially buried in the ground beside the skulls. There were no marks on the bones and I assumed that they had not died violent deaths. I was not going to disturb their remains by digging about, yet I couldn't stop wondering how and when the bones got there. The skulls could be father and child. Indian? Not likely. The natives in the north, when they are not copying our customs, bury their dead on high ridges, each grave with some kind of fence or covering. If they are close to a town they often build little houses over the graves complete with windows, eating utensils and other objects. I looked around but could find no trace of a cabin or home. It was an unlikely place for a cabin in any case for cabins were usually built in valleys near fuel and water.

The problems of finding shelter in the bush had intrigued me since I had come north and I tried to re-create the history of some of the old cabins I saw. Most old cabins rot from the roof down, possibly because the logs close to the ground are so close to the permafrost. Wood lasts a long time in the Yukon for nothing rots in the frigid cold of the eight-month winter. I saw cedar shingles brought to Dawson in the eighteen-nineties that were still in fair shape fifty years later. I particularly liked exploring old cabin sites marked only by a clearing left after a fire. In addition to the gap in the forest you could usually see three pieces of evidence. First, a tumble-down outhouse could usually be found nearby. Second, there was often a thriving patch of rhubarb near the cabin site, planted decades before by the original miner or trapper and third, there was usually a patch of delphiniums, native or imported, still flowering near the cabin.

But back to the skulls. If not those of Indians, the skulls could have been of early Russian trappers or explorers who had died and been buried by their friends in the shallow graves. To this day, the skeletons still rest in that lonely spot. The flowers and the squaw-berries still grow out of the holes in their skulls ready to teach a passer-by the same lesson that the Irish poet Yeats ordered to be inscribed on his head-stone:

> *Cast a cold eye*
> *On life, on death.*
> *Horseman, pass by!*

I had my own brush with death soon after I walked back to my friends' truck. It had been moved close to an unused cabin a short distance off the road and my friends had been joined by several men living in a shed across the valley. I was told that they were prospecting with a bulldozer. Everyone had gone to bed in the old bunks away from the opening where the door used to be and I bunked down in my sleeping bag across the door opening. When my eyes became accustomed to the semi-light I saw that the men were sleeping with their rifles at their sides but thought nothing of it. In the morning I learned that a large grizzly bear had broken into the prospectors' shed the previous day and had prowled about all evening, forcing them out. They had decided it was safer to sleep in the old cabin. I had slept soundly, not realizing that my position across the door put me first in line to become a victim for the marauding bear.

SICK HORSE, BRAVE MOOSE

Not enough wonder drug

Sometimes I was asked to treat sick horses for they were very valuable in Dawson. The horses were chiefly used for hauling the wood for kitchen stoves and furnaces. Late in January one year Dr. Geoff Homer and I were asked to go over to the red light district to see a sick mare. When we got to the stable John Gannon, the local amateur veterinarian, told us that a big Clydesdale mare had "black-water fever". He based his diagnosis on the fact that she was passing only small amounts of dark urine. Gannon was convinced that if she could void the illness would be cured. Gannon said he would have no problem with a male horse since he definitely knew where the penis was and could put in a catheter easily. But this was a mare and he didn't know where to put the catheter. He figured that mares were probably built like women and since we were experts in that field we ought to be able to help the mare.

Gannon's diagnosis did not make much sense to us but we decided to do what he wanted. Our catheters would be too small and Geoff suggested that a stomach tube would be about right for our over-sized patient. A large one was brought from the hospital, boiled up and well-lubricated. Our first attempt was almost a disaster. When we approached her rear, the mare, sensing some hanky-panky, lashed out. She missed us but broke several two by fours. We tied her up and managed to insert the catheter. Production? Only a few drops of concentrated urine. Gannon then decided that production of urine could be stimulated by hot packs (bags of warm salt tied to her back.) We did not wait for the results of this treatment because it was obvious the mare was dying of pneumonia. At that time a sulfa drug, M&B 693, was available for pneumonia but there was not enough in town to be of any use to such a large patient and so we walked home sadly in the bitter cold.

Way to kill wolves

Henry LeBlanc was a clever trapper who lived at Gravel Lake outside Dawson, famed for killing timber wolves by an ingenious method he had invented. LeBlanc would get a thigh bone of a moose or caribou, remove the marrow and melt it, mix it with strychnine and then replace the mixture in the bone. The bone was then stuck upright like a fence post in the thick lake ice. Attracted by the bone's scent, the wolves would gnaw on the strychnine-laced marrow and quickly die in convulsions, usually close by the bone. LeBlanc would then cut off the ears and collect the bounty. This method was outlawed later because the entrails of the poisoned wolves were eaten by other carnivora, foxes and wolverines. Even birds like the large Arctic ravens eventually became victims to LeBlanc's strychnine.

So he found another way to kill wolves. When he was young and living in Quebec LeBlanc had been an excellent skater and hockey player. In the Yukon there is a short time in the late fall when the lakes are firmly frozen but not covered by snow. Henry used to enjoy skating at this time and noticed that the wolves could not walk properly on the ice. He had found a new way of killing the animals! One night LeBlanc dragged a batch of moose and cariboo entrails onto the lake ice to attract the wolves. The next morning he donned skates and moved out to meet the surprised wolf pack. Running away, they began skidding and slipping on the ice—easy targets for Henry.

Tough old moose

My friend Johnny Hoggan, a dredge-master for Consolidated Gold Corporation in Dawson, told me he that he saw an incredible battle between a bear and a bull moose. Hoggan was walking along a ridge high up in the Klondyke river watershed when he heard crashing in the willow scrub below. He cleared a path and saw a grizzly fighting a bull moose. The bear would charge the moose then rear up on his hind legs and slash at the chest of the moose with his powerful front paws. The bear's head and neck were then exposed to the kicks from the razor-sharp hooves of the moose. The bear fell back after each charge to all four feet and allowed the moose to get more kicks into the grizzly's head. Eventually, the bear appeared to have gone blind, for he just lay there while the moose tore his body to pieces with his antlers and

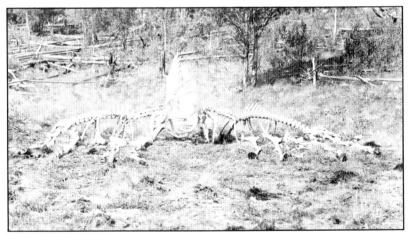

Moose locked in combat starve to death

hooves. The moose moved slowly away. His chest was ripped bare to the ribs; neck bleeding; and his antlers broken. The grizzly is one of the biggest, meanest and strongest animals in the world yet this moose had killed him. He was badly wounded and so Hoggan put him to sleep with one shot from his 30-30 rifle. The moose's scarred haunches told of many battles with wolf packs. If his off-spring inherited his courage the wolves would have no easy pickings.

HOSPITAL LIFE

First, take in the laundry

Everything worked well at the Dawson hospital except the wretched, old-fashioned X-ray machine. Power for the X-ray tube came from a five-foot wheel rotated by an electric motor. On the outer edge of the wheel were pads of a furry material that rotated rapidly against glass pads. The whirling wheel accumulated static electricity. When the voltage was large enough it emitted a startling bolt of lightning across two knob-like electrodes. That was the signal to throw the charge into the tube taking the X-ray picture. On damp days it was difficult to get the voltage high enough to take a picture, for the static electricity would not build up when the humidity was high. This cranky old machine was used only for fractures and other coarse readings because the pictures were so poor. But who was not impressed by the display of the flashing electrodes! This ancient rig used over-head cables from the static accumulator to the X-ray tube. When not in use these cables served as laundry lines for the nurses' underwear and so the first item in taking an X-ray picture was to gather in the laundry. Later, about 1940, we got a modern portable machine.

Practice for surgery

The lower floor of the hospital was filled with elderly men, most of whom were blind or partially blind. They were pioneers who had come to Dawson during the gold rush, failed to find, or keep, their fortune and had stayed in the Yukon. Most of them had cataracts and were almost blind but they did not have enough money to go south for surgery. I had learned some basic ophthalmology but I wasn't trained to remove cataracts. So in 1938, en route to Florida on vacation, my wife and I arranged to stay at the Mayo Clinic in Rochester to watch cataract surgery. Every morning for ten days I watched the eye surgeons at work. Then, when I got back to Dawson, I asked the hospital to buy the instruments I needed. They soon arrived, even a Smith cataract knife, a fearful-looking knife curved like a scimitar.

A little practice before using these instruments seemed in order. Cariboo eyes seemed just the thing, large and plentiful and an order was placed with a puzzled Indian friend. He arrived with a pail-full and I began to use them for practice surgery. About a week later a group of Indian women arrived with a basket of meat. They explained that they were sorry I was reduced to eating cariboo eyes and deserved better cuts.

My first cataract patient was Dan Stears, a good-natured man, almost blind. I chose his left eye for a very good reason—the nose would not be in the way for a right-handed surgeon. The fixation forceps held the eye steady and, with some trepidation, I pushed the knife across the cornea. Everything went well and two minutes later the eye looked clear and clean. "My God, Doc," said Stears, "I can see the lights in the ceiling."

After the corneal wound had healed we needed to get some glasses for Dan so that he could read with his good eye. We used an old testing frame and got a satisfactory refraction. Then we put in a spare testing lens to make him a set of spectacles, for he could not afford to buy any and we had no money for such things. After our success with Stears, we did a few more cataract operations. Some were failures because the retina had deteriorated before surgery, but I do not remember ever losing two eyes in any man. I was thrilled a few months later to see Stears reading a newspaper at the Christmas party given for the old men. He looked up and said "Thank you, doctor, for my best-ever Christmas present. I was blind and now I can see."

Blood for a murderer

It was a cold, raw, blustery day in early spring. The snow in Dawson was melting in little dirty patches. The phone rang in my office in the hospital. "Better come down to the Yukon Hotel, Doc," said a deep, calm voice, "there's a guy down here in trouble." My car started easily for a change—thanks to the warming spring sun—and I set out to the Yukon Hotel, an old two-storey log building right across from the Anglican Church. It dated back to the gold rush days and its floors were uneven due to the heaving and thawing of its permafrost base. Now it was being used as a hostel for transients.

I parked my car beside the church and walked over to the front of the hotel. There was nobody around. A team of horses was hitched to a load of wood standing near the hotel entrance. Then I saw a man lying on the ground in front of the horses with his head almost entirely blown off. There was a huge pool of blood around him. Before I could get my wits together, a Mountie stuck his head out of an upper-storey window and said, "Don't bother with that guy, he's dead. Come up and see the one up here. He's still alive." In a front bedroom, I found a man trying to wash blood from a space that used to be occupied by his lower jaw, mouth and most of his upper jaw. He had shot the wood dealer whose body was lying in the street and then tried to shoot himself. But he had pointed the rifle forward when he put it under his chin instead of backwards and had blown away his lower face.

Since he was still on his feet, we stuffed a towel in the wound and walked him down to my car and rushed him to the hospital. We had just got our first supplies of a new intravenous anaesthetic called Evipal, a precursor of the Pentothal that is still used today. Evipal was slowly injected into an arm vein whereas our usual anaesthetic was ether by inhalation mask over the nose and mouth. This man had neither, so we had to use Evipal. As soon as he went to sleep we did the best we could to repair his face, sewing together any remaining viable pieces and controlling bleeding. To help him breathe we put a tube in his windpipe but to save his life we needed lots of blood. For years the Mounties had been our chief source of blood. Of course, we had no laboratory to properly match blood for transfusions, so I simply made a direct match between the donor and the patient.

Years earlier I had read that in an emergency you could give blood safely without full laboratory examination through a procedure called Coco's method. All you needed was a little chloroform and those small pipettes we used in counting the cells in a patients' blood. A small volume of whole donor's blood was mixed with a relatively large volume of a recipient's blood serum. You prepared this by treating the whole blood with a little chloroform. This dissolved the red cells of the recipient blood and produced serum. When you mixed grossly incompatible bloods you could see clumps of clotted cells appearing with the naked eye. A look through a microscope easily spotted less obvious incompatibilities.

And so we asked for donors for the murderer but there were no volunteers. One constable summed it all up. "Why the hell save him now," he asked, "just to hang him later?" The man died a few days later without regaining consciousness.

Follow the swallow

One of our most interesting patients was a tall, thin French Canadian from Gravel Lake who was slowly starving to death. His English was rather limited and since I only understood high school French it took some time to learn what was wrong. After several attempts to communicate he asked me for a glass of water. I gave it to him and he swallowed it. I noticed that his neck began to swell. Then, after pushing me back to clear the decks, he squeezed his neck with his hands and squirted out the water. This showed his problem better than a thousand words: his food and drink was getting trapped in his throat.

I gave him an X-ray with a barium swallow and this showed that he had a very large pouch leading off his lower throat. It was so large that any swallowed material ran into this sac instead of down to his stomach - much like a squirrel packing nuts. The books all said the only treatment was surgery so surgery it had to be.

I had to go through the left side of his neck, in front of the large blood vessels and behind the voice-box and wind-pipe. I had never been in this neck area before; the nearest was rather lower when I was removing a goitrous thyroid. When I reached the gullet I could see the pouch behind it, like a hernia sac and the size of a small tangerine orange. What next? It was tempting to cut it off, sewing over the stump, but this was before antibiotics. Infection from the opened throat could go down into his chest. I decided to pull the sac up and tuck it under the jaw at the upper end of the incision. Food and fluids would then run down to his stomach by gravity with little effort by the patient. If this did not happen we could go back in a week or ten days after adhesions had formed when it would be safer to remove the sac.

The wound was drained and when he came round I explained my plan to the patient. He agreed but was soon demanding that he be allowed to try to swallow. To my amazement water sailed down into his stomach very easily. Then we tried soups and solid food—all slid down readily past the elevated and now-fixed pouch. My skinny patient rapidly grew into a tubby patient without a second operation, something we were all happy to omit in that pre-sulfa and pre-penicillin age.

Tricky toy

I had another unusual neck surgery case a few months later. The patient was a little Indian girl who had been playing with a toy called a jack. This blunt spiked metal object is spun on one of its legs, later coming to rest on the remaining legs. This girl had put it in her mouth and swallowed it. The legs twisted and, acting like flukes on a sea anchor, became firmly secured in her gullet at the level of the voice box.

In most hospitals removing the jack would be relatively easy, using a special pair of forceps with a light attached, but we had nothing like that around. I waited a day or two. X-rays, however, showed the anchored jack was not about to move and the throat was becoming swollen. This could interfere with the girl's breathing and made surgery imperative. I opened the neck on the left side as I did for the man with the neck pouch. I felt where the jack was, opened the gullet, took it out and sutured the wound in the gullet. The neck wound was only lightly sutured with several soft drains. No serious infection developed and the girl was back at school in two weeks.

Fore-skins for grafts

Charlie Roberts was a young Indian who got second- and third-degree burns to his arms, chest and back when a fire broke out in his cabin. In hospital we cleaned him up and removed the loose skin and tried to make him comfortable. But the day after he had been admitted his circulation started to collapse because he had lost so much fluid from his burns. I found that his blood was very concentrated, almost sticky. These days everyone is aware of this problem but I had never encountered it before. His heart could not cope with the sticky blood and we quickly started to drip some saline solution into his veins. It took nearly six litres to lower the concentration of his blood to a safe level.

Charlie had a stormy convalescence because he needed extensive skin-grafts. I first covered raw areas with skin taken from his legs. Then, when I had used up all the available part of his legs, I tried using the baby sacs from our maternity patients. I even used the fore-skins from circumcised babies, splitting the skin into layers. All this snipping and grafting made Charlie very depressed. I am afraid that I am not much good at psychiatric counselling but I got help from a strange place—the ventilator hole in his room. A pair of bluebirds had made their nest in the hole and their chirping and rustling as they raised a family gave Charlie the courage to survive.

A few stitches too many

It was the fall of 1939. The temperature was well below freezing; the rivers were running bank to bank with blocks of ice; and the gold dredges were shutting down for the season. The dredge on Upper Sulphur Creek was bucking ice in her self-made pond, inching forward to get a good resting spot for the winter, when a member of the crew, Chris Bredenberg fell into the tail-run of waste rock and was carried over the stacker. His arm was torn off at the shoulder and he was bleeding profusely. Geoff Homer and I left Dawson as soon as we got the telephone call. It was pitch dark, snowing lightly and the driver of our pickup truck decided to take a short cut though a rarely-used side road. As we climbed a hill we saw that an old truck had been abandoned in the middle of the road. We got out, went to the nearest cabin and found that it belonged to a deaf and dumb machinist who serviced pumps and hoists in Dawson. He had parked his truck there for the winter and didn't want to move it! We had no time to waste and so pushed the truck off the edge of the road and down into a small gully.

When we reached the dredge we found Bredenberg on a repair bench. He was covered with blankets. Blood was everywhere. His severed arm had been placed on a blanket by his side. When we looked in the gaping hole at the shoulder we could see the remains of the shattered head of the arm bone. The large arm artery had retracted well up into the arm pit and the fact that his arm had been pulled off, rather than cut, had probably saved his life. If it had been severed by something sharp he would have bled to death before we could reach him.

We took him back to the hospital in the pick-up. The nurses got him cleaned up, warmed up and then started an intravenous with our home-made saline solution. But that only replaced fluids. We needed blood and got some that matched from an RCMP officer. Later, under ether anaesthesia, we cleaned up the wound and trimmed the flaps of skin. Then I made the mistake that almost cost Chris his life. The wound looked so neat and clean that I put in a few stitches to tidy it up. Not many, but too many. Geoff warned me about closure. We both were aware of the danger of gangrene. Chris did very well for a few days, but then one morning I smelled the pungent smell of gas gangrene as I came to his bed. As I probed into the wound I could hear the peculiar crackling sound of gas in the tissue. Immediately we moved Chris out of the ward into the basement to avoid infecting the other patients and took out the stitches. But the wound was already giving off a typical pink, smelly discharge and all the muscles of the chest wall came away until only the ribs were left.

He seemed to recover at first but in a few days he got worse. We gave him all the gas gangrene anti-serum we had without effect. I had read that X-ray radiation was useful in gas gangrene so our diagnostic machine was lined up and used. The dose? Just the maximum advised for regular work—but it also had no effect on Chris's condition. We thought we were going to lose him until we remembered our ace in the hole. Some months before we had used a new drug called sulfanilamide to treat gonorrhoea, pelvic disease and assorted traumatic infections. Our preparation, called Prontosil, worked very well. But in gas gangrene? We had never heard of its use in this infection but we had no choice and so Geoff and I decided to use it. The Prontosil worked like a miracle and Bredenberg survived to live out his normal life.

Alcohol the cure

One summer day a gaunt, unshaven man came into my waiting room, took a seat and silently waited until I was free. He told me he had travelled to Dawson by a small river boat from his cabin about ten miles downstream and was a trapper and miner. His lower jaw hung open, saliva trickled over his chin, and he spoke only in a whisper for it was difficult for him to move his tongue. He told me that he had suffered with bouts of severe pain in his left cheek for several years. The pain was getting worse and he often thought that suicide was the only way out. Painkillers did not work for him any more and he wanted me to help him. He had a bad case of tic douloureux and for a while I treated him with alcohol injections of the cheek nerve. These gave him relief from the pain for months at a time but after a while it was obvious that he would need an alcohol block of the nerve at the skull base. Some years ago I had helped a neuro-surgeon do this with good results and so I decided to do it on this poor man.

To reach the nerve a long hollow needle was introduced through the side of his face to a hole in the skull base called the rotundum (round) that carried the nerve. This had to be done with only a local anaesthetic because the patient had to tell us when we had hit the source of his pain. After we had found this spot I injected Evipal into his arm and he immediately fell asleep. Then I injected alcohol through the pre-positioned needle. He was in shock for a while but was then free of pain for years.

Eventually a proper neuro-surgeon operated on him and the pain never came back.

Death comes close

With all its antiquated equipment and lack of skilled staff to help the doctor the hospital was still the best place to perform even minor operations.

Early one wintry morning the phone rang in my home and a man's voice asked me to go to see a sick Indian girl who lived in the northern part of the town. I put on my coon coat and walked through the drifting snow for about half a mile before I came to a sad-looking shack. Pieces of newspaper had been stuffed into cracks in the walls and broken window panes. Inside, children of various ages peered at me from old boxes, piles of clothes and bunks. On one bunk lay my patient, obviously very ill. Her dark eyes stared at me from under a thatch of black hair. She looked about six years old and her mother said she was feverish, had a sore throat and could not swallow anything.

The lymph glands under her jaw were swollen and when I looked into her mouth with my flashlight I could see that her tonsils were very enlarged. Under the left one was a large quinsy, a collection of pus that practically blocked her throat. The quinsy had to be drained. I put the little girl on her side and injected a few drops of Novocaine into the tip of the swelling. Then, with her father holding the light, I made a small cut in the anaesthetised area. No pus came out. I gave her a little more Novocaine and since I did not want to deepen the cut and risk a haemorrhage, I poked the tip of a pair of artery forceps into the incision—with almost disastrous results. A mass of pus spurted out and ran down her throat. The little girl choked and turned blue. Luckily she was small and so I picked her up and shook her and the bloody pus flowed out of her mouth. She breathed with a gasp and was alright.

I now realised that she had a large abscess that had been hidden by the quinsy and that I should have taken her to hospital where I could have operated on a table that tilted her head down. She was soon running about as if nothing had ever been wrong.

DANGERS OF BIRTH

In favor of Caesareans

Some people probably think that delivering babies was the easiest task I had to perform in the North. That simply wasn't so. The threat of disaster frequently loomed large over the delivery table and if the mother was injured I would lose much of the confidence of the community. A fracture can be poorly set; a herniotomy be a failure; haemorrhoids can return; but who can forgive the doctor when a full-term baby is still-born? And it's worse if the mother is lost. Remember that I was usually the only doctor and so all blame was directed at me. It is true that most babies arrive safely without much attention from anybody. In fact a minimum of interference makes for good obstetrics. Many times a good long walk, leaving the laboring mother with a capable nurse, results upon one's return in an easy delivery instead of forceps. Still, there is always the very real chance of haemorrhage, vomiting food under anaesthetic, pressure on the umbilical cord or an embolus (a blood clot impeding the circulation).

In the Yukon I delivered over three hundred babies and this

figure does not include the babies born to Indian women I attended in their homes when there was an emergency. Whenever there were problems I remembered that there was always the possibility of a Caesarean. If there is obstructed labour and a Caesarean isn't possible you have to perform difficult and complicated manoeuvres or use high forceps—often damaging the babies' heads and causing horrendous tears to the mothers. I used Caesarean section whenever prolonged labour resulted in no progress—no matter what the cause. When there was haemorrhage or placenta previa (after-birth ahead of the baby) it was the only way out, even if I had to do the sections in the back-woods, without antibiotics, emergency blood or skilled assistance.

Messy childbirth

Often deliveries were merely messy and not at all interesting. Once I was called to see an Indian woman who was in protracted labour. The only nurse who was available to help was all dressed up in a fur coat and a nice dress but she agreed to come with me. Indian women prefer to deliver their babies sitting on the floor so that they can press their feet against a box that has been nailed to the floor. Pushing against the box helps press the baby out; not a bad idea, for sitting up is better than lying down to get the baby's head moving. Our patient was doing just that when we arrived but the well-dressed nurse had never done floor deliveries before and she tried to move the woman so that I could deliver the head and free the cord if necessary. As the baby's head started to move, the woman's bladder let go a half-day's accumulation of urine. Then her bowels did their stuff. The amniotic fluid was then added to the mess and into this mixture out popped a black head of hair—the baby. The nurse was filthy but game and we tied the cord well away from the baby to avoid infection. Finally the afterbirth came out and added blood to the messy mixture. We washed the baby, took it to the hospital and, as usual, it did fine. As a final indignity the nurse found lice in her clothes the next day.

Even when they came to hospital Indian women often refused to lie in bed to deliver their babies. One day I went into the labor room and saw a nurse chasing an Indian woman who was running around the room with her baby's head partially out. The nurse had to hold a sheet to catch the baby and wrestle the mother into a bed at the same time.

Permanently pregnant

In those days many Indian women seemed to have been pregnant all their lives. After delivering a baby they seldom had time to menstruate before another pregnancy was on the way. This sometimes resulted in the woman dying of uterine inertia if the baby was not delivered by Caesarean section or forceps. The first Caesarean section ever performed in Mayo was made on an Indian woman with fourteen babies who just could not deliver her baby because of uterine inertia. If I hadn't operated the mother would have died from infection or haemorrhage. And many Indian women fifty years ago had severe rickets when they were young. This often resulted in a deformed pelvis and obstructed delivery. Caesarean section was the only way to save mother and child.

Problem premies

The handling of premature babies posed a special problem for we did not have incubators. The Dawson nurses solved this problem by devising a method that worked very well.

Mrs. Olga Nelson's premie, a little girl, was about the size of a loaf of bread when she was born. The nurses packed her in absorbent cotton with only her little puckered face showing. This packing kept her warm and could be changed to clean her up. I suspect the nurses got the idea from seeing how the Indian women kept their babies in moss-filled sacks on boards strapped to their backs. The next problem was food. Fortunately, we had several mothers breast-feeding their own babies in the hospital and the little girl was fed their milk through an eye dropper. She was kept in a clothes basket in the centre of the hospital corridor and people passing by would give her a squirt, assuring she got a good supply of milk. Oxygen? We had none, fortunately, for without any way of measuring the oxygen concentration, we would have risked scarring the baby's eyes. She grew up to be a normal little girl.

Family planning?

The arrival of babies continually disrupted my plans to go hunting, especially since the fall open season on moose was so short. So I wrote a short notice to be published in the local paper nine months before hunting season opened. It went like this: "Dawson residents are respectfully requested to avoid conception in the month of December, so the doctor can go hunting next fall." But Harold Malstom, the worldly-wise editor of the Dawson News, just snorted when I brought it in and said, "Forget it and save the price of the ad." He was right. December nights were long and cold in Dawson and my chance of changing the pattern of life there was nil.

Paternal participation

In my last year at Dawson the idea that a father should watch his child's arrival had become fairly common. It was new to me—and not a good idea, either, for we had enough troubles without having an anxious male around.

We tried to dissuade paternal participation in the birth process but one man insisted. He turned up just before the baby was born. The mother had been sedated with a form of anaesthesia called "twilight sleep" that made her confused and not the least bit cheery about the whole painful performance. After a very difficult contraction, the father tried to console his wife. She looked up through her stupor and said, "Get the hell out of here, you hypocrite. If it weren't for you I wouldn't be in this position now." And that ended our trial of having fathers observe the results of their handiwork.

Tiny transfusion

George Berg was our orderly and X-Ray technician and so we paid special attention when his wife Netta had twins. The delivery presented no problem, but both babies were very pale and we had no idea what the trouble was. It may have been RH incompatibility but at that time we knew nothing about it. Very soon the babies were very weak and one of them died. The second baby was also about to die when we decided to try and save him with a transfusion. There were two problems: whose blood to use and how could we get blood into this tiny body?

We gambled on the father as the donor. There was a good chance of his being compatible and so we checked his blood by Coco's method directly with the baby's. It matched. Then we opened a vein in his tiny arm and under local anaesthesia managed to get a canula into a vein. We made the canula by filing the sharp end of a syringe needle until it was smooth and round. Then George's blood was cautiously injected into his son. The baby gradually turned pink and, with the help of another transfusion next day, recovered to become a normal child.

INDIAN LIFE

Keeping warm at 60 below

The Department of Indian Affairs was, in effect, one of my
employers while I was in the Yukon and I was expected to
provide medical care to the Indians in the areas close to where I
worked. About a third of my patients were Indians and they
belonged to the Loucheux bands which are believed to have
originated in Asia. Their facial characteristics, such as the epi-
canthic fold over the corner of their eyes, were of the Mongolian
type. And most of them had RH negative blood, similar to
Asians; the reverse proportion is found in whites and prairie
Indians. The Indians, as I knew them in the Thirties, were very
different from the present generation. In Mayo, where my first
contacts were made, the whole tribe or groups of families would
arrive in town from the far north. Most of them were nomads
from the Peel River, the Old Crow area and the Mackenzie Delta.
They came only in the winter, for travel was impossible over the
marshy ground in the summer.

They were dressed almost wholly in the skins of the animals
they caught and they designed their clothes to protect themselves

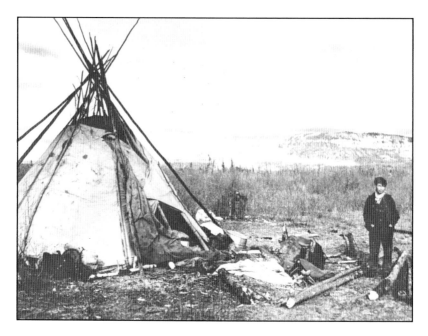

Indian home: some canvas and poles

from temperatures that could reach 60 below for weeks on end. At this temperature merely the movement of their sleigh could cause enough wind to increase the wind chill factor substantially. On the outside both men and women wore a loose-fitting, rough parka made usually from cariboo or moose hide. This garment had to be loose to permit free striding in walking, running or riding a sled but snug at the neck to trap the body heat collected in the lower bell-like part. Indian women sewed the tailored skins together with thread made from the teased-out fibres of the cariboo's Achilles tendon. They had to cut the opening in the parka's hood so that the face was protected from the wind and snow and yet allow the wearer to see where she or he was going. The opening was always lined with wolverine fur for the Indians had learned long ago that this fur did not frost up with the wearer's breath. Without the protective hood one's eyelids froze together; the eyeballs ached, and breathing caused pains in the chest, especially breathing through the mouth. Trousers of a lighter cariboo skin completed the outer clothes for both men and women. Underwear was made from the skins of unborn cariboo or moose and worn with the down-like hair next to the body for extra warmth. The women's bloomers were the biggest I have ever seen. One summer we had several Indian women in the Mayo hospital at the same time and the clothes line was loaded with their bloomers, blowing in the wind like spinnakers.

The feet were covered by loose moccasins, usually made of moose-hide and tanned with wood-ash. These were worn very loose and made their wearer's feet look like legs of mutton. But they were very warm and few Indians had frost-bitten feet if they were wearing these moccasins. Usually the moccasin was extended to form a mukluk which was tied at the knee.

Children wore junior versions of these clothes. Babies were tucked into a moose-skin sack mounted on a board and then the space around them was packed with lichen. In most parts of the Yukon the "ground" was really a layer of lichen over the permafrost. The Indian women collected this and dried it in large heaps inside their tents. This packing not only kept the baby warm but was absorbent and so served as a quickly replaceable diaper. It was always surprising to me how clean this kept the babies, for they had few skin problems. It was certainly much better than poorly-laundered cloth diapers.

Home-grown sunglasses

Every spring the Indians had to cope, like everybody else, with snow blindness. The early spring sun, reflected at a low angle off the clean snow, rapidly causes painful eye inflammation and blindness if the eyes are not protected. The Indians learned long ago how to cope with this problem by looking through a slit in a piece of bone. The shoulder blade of a cariboo has a very thin area near the centre of the bone. The Indians removed part of this piece of bone, fashioned it into a crude pair of spectacles and carefully cut a narrow horizontal slit in front of each eye.

Sex and the sun

The early spring sun in the sub-Arctic must contain a spectrum of rays different from more southerly areas. I had often noticed how this spring sun stimulated plant growth. Radishes, lettuce, and tomatoes seemed to rush to maturity. Not so the September sun, even if in quantity it equalled the April sun. There must surely be a qualitative difference. The April sun affected not only plants but also birds, animals and humans.

Years ago, Jack Miner studied migrating Canada geese at his Ontario bird sanctuary. Why, he asked, do geese go north in the spring, south in the fall? He irradiated the heads of a few geese in the late fall and the birds insisted upon mating and flying north in freezing weather. He concluded that the pituitary glands in the birds' heads were probably stimulated by the gamma radiation, initiating sex and northern migration. Whatever the cause the spring sun did remarkable things to people as well as plants and birds. For years I had noticed that I grew more intolerant as winter advanced. I even began to hate the way our neighbors—all nice people—walked. It was especially hard on women, both Indian and white, cooped up with children in the cold Arctic darkness. Then the sun came. Suddenly, we all became tolerant and happy once more and, best of all, came a fringe benefit—a revival of sexual interest. The arrival of the sun seemed to affect most Yukoners, both Indian and white, who lived in the outdoors substantially and I was told that this sexual cycle particularly affected Eskimos and others living in the High Arctic. There were, I am sure, no unhappy maidens in the northern springtime.

Labour-saving, Indian style

The Indians I knew were not worry-warts. They did not worry about tomorrow, nor did they do unnecessary work. Consider their tents, their homes. When cold weather came they simply put a second tent over the primary summer tent, insulating it from snow and frost. Wood? Why cut and stack a large pile? The easiest way was to get a long dry log and progressively shove it into the stove; no sawing needed. In addition the log was an excellent seat, automatically warmed as it neared the stove. On the floor they stacked spruce boughs; soft to sleep upon and a place for the children to play. On occasion while visiting an Indian family in their tent, I was surprised to find a little, black-haired head pop up among the boughs on the floor.

Then there's this example: our house in Dawson had a six-foot side-walk from the porch to the street board-walk. The city kept this clear of snow with a horse-drawn plow but it was up to me to shovel our short stretch. Almost every morning after the night's wind and snow I shovelled the walk. Inevitably, as the banks got deeper, the snow blew in again. One of our Indian neighbours walked past our house each morning on his way to work in the power-house and noticed my ineffective shovelling. Finally, he could stand it no longer. He stopped, watched me shovel snow into the wind, and said, "White man crazy like hell. All winter you shovel snow; wind blows it back again; soon comes the sun; snow melts. You crazy like hell!"

But then there's this: An Indian boy had been injured at Wellesley Lake, a hundred miles to the south, and the Department of Indian Affairs sent me there by plane. Unfortunately, the boy had died before we got there and we decided to wait a few hours before taking off for Dawson because the smoke from a forest fire filled the sky. Tied to the shore was a crude raft made of several water-soaked logs. Having noticed fish jumping in the

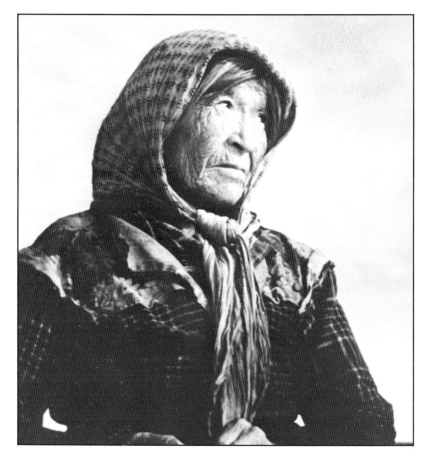

Indian woman. Photo by Ted Field

lake, I persuaded an old Indian man to paddle me out to the raft so that I could try my luck casting. (I usually took my fishing-gear with me in the summer.) After practically every cast I caught a fish, mostly large northern pike. My guide did not want these bony fish, for the Indians at the lake had barrels of white-fish, a much tastier fish, caught by the hundreds in nets. And so I had fun catching pike for dog feed. When I got to shore I asked why the tribe did not smoke or salt some of the whitefish for winter use. They replied, "Why bother? White man always worries about what comes next." And they had no salt. Furthermore, the cariboo would be back in the fall to fill the larder. Anyway, they were tired of fish!

In the afternoon the smoke had lifted and in an hour we were back in Dawson. Four months later we had to air-lift food to the Indians at Wellesley Lake. They were starving. The cariboo migration had failed.

TB the killer

Tuberculosis was an unmitigated disaster for the Indians. Some families had private cemeteries in their backyards filled with the bodies of children and young adults who had died from the disease. It was so virulent that many children never lived long enough to develop the usual pulmonary forms, for the infection acted as an acute disease with tuberculous meningitis as the immediate cause of death. One winter, during a holiday outside, I went to the Fort Qu'Appelle Sanitorium in Saskatchewan for several weeks to learn about treatment of TB. The "rest" treatment was ineffective and not practical in the Yukon for we had no facilities for prolonged rest in bed. Besides, how could nomads be accommodated? For several years I tried the lung-collapse techniques that I learned at Qu'Appelle but the results were very poor. Happily, with the new antibiotics and better hospital facilities TB is disappearing in the North.

Death is the final sleep

The Indians I met were used to death and dying. They saw it daily as they slaughtered and trapped animals for their livelihood. For them everything had its time, ending in death, and they could not understand our fear of dying. "Why do white people fear death?" they often asked me. "Nobody fears the onset of the unconsciousness called sleep yet you are afraid of the final sleep, death."

DAWSON PEOPLE

The Yukon had so many things to offer a doctor in the Thirties and Forties. The opportunity to practice a frontier brand of medicine was one; the close contact with nature was another. But perhaps the best of all was being able to meet so many wonderful and colorful people. Here are a few I knew in Dawson:

Gum-boot McLeod

He got his name because it was rare to see him wearing any other foot-wear. He was a hero in my eyes because he died in a way I have always admired. He had cancer of the stomach and we told him that surgery was useless and that he would die shortly. He accepted this gracefully and set his house in order. His loving and attentive wife looked after him. I visited him regularly and he never complained but became weaker and, after a short farewell, died in peace. No fuss, no nonsense, just the last chapter and a lesson in how to die with dignity.

Rubber-neck Johnson

Jim Johnson was our post-master. He had injured his neck when he was young and kept it at an angle—hence his nickname. Johnson was a celebrated hockey player in Dawson's early days. He was the enforcer and had a crooked nose to show for it. Johnson was big-hearted, a feared poker player and a master-drinker of rum. He taught me both of these pastimes and they stood me in good stead during my Yukon tenure.

Christmas is drinking time

John MacLennon was Dawson's druggist and a former Mountie. His store was downtown and he stocked a good supply of drugs for a small place like Dawson; in addition he'd get anything the hospital asked him for. John was also my landlord and the floors above his store bore a sign that read: The Dawson Medical Dental Building. Dr. Irving E. Snider, Dentist. Dr. Allan Duncan, MD. MacLennon had one serious fault. He drank himself stupid in the week between Christmas and New Year's Day. For the rest of the year he was teetotal but as Christmas came around, John said, he itched all over and had to have alcohol. Unfortunately there was sixty below zero weather at that time of the year and when John drank nothing else mattered; so every Christmas his friends had to keep John's fires going to prevent his pipes and stock from freezing. We also tried cross-threading the bung of his little barrel of pharmaceutical alcohol but he always got the alcohol out somehow.

Habits die hard

Irving Snider stayed in Dawson for the summer months, and he and his partner were the faithful custodians of Yukon teeth for many years. They arrived on the first spring boat and left at freeze-up. Most of Snider's dentistry was done at mining camps where there was no electricity or running water. He had a portable, canvas dental chair and a foot-treadle to generate power for his drill. Recently in Vancouver, when he was touching up some inlays he had put in my teeth fifty years earlier, I looked down from his magnificent modern dental chair and, sure enough, as soon as the high speed turbo-drill was put in my mouth, Snider's foot started pumping, a reflex he hadn't lost. Snider's inlays were built to last: I can still crack nuts with the gold anvils he put in my molars in the Yukon.

Berton - the sailor

When Irving Snider was away Frank Berton used to pull many an aching tooth. My predecessor had left him some dental instruments and Berton used his mechanical skill to good advantage on decayed teeth. Berton was the Gold Commissioner during most of my stay in Dawson. He was a kind, interesting man who lived a few doors down Seventh Avenue from our house. His son, Pierre, is the famous writer.

Berton had a winter hobby—grinding optical glass to make telescope mirrors. During the summer, however, Berton loved his boat and spent many weekends boating on the Yukon River. Unfortunately we never could persuade him to take enough replacement shear pins for his outboard motor, essential because the river was full of wind-falls and other flotsam. If the accident occurred up-stream, Berton could float home; if it was downstream, we had to go out and rescue him.

At Christmas, we often asked men whose family was "outside" to come to dinner with us. Berton was one of these. He was an entertaining guest and was a favorite of our children.

Teasing a bear

One bright summer day my wife admitted a man called Len Sharples into our parlour. I was at work in another room and so could hear only snatches of their conversation. It went something like this: My wife: "She chased you up a tree, did she? My, she must have been mad at you!" Sharples: "You might say that." My wife: "She really bit your toes off. My, you must have been teasing her!" My curiosity was aroused and I went into the parlour. There was Sharples sitting there holding three toes and a piece of his boot neatly amputated by a bear that had treed him. I soon had Sharples' foot stitched up but couldn't do anything for his boot.

Wedding surprise

Rev. Creighton McCullum and Rev. Jack Vance were the ministers in charge of the Anglican churches in Mayo and Dawson. In both towns all the Protestants went to the Anglican church and both McCullum and Vance asked me to be Rector's warden, in spite of my Presbyterian background. One of my duties in both towns was to take up the collection in a little bag on the end of a stick. Each Sunday I canvassed the congregation and choir with my bag and stick but the "take" was poor from the choir until I learned the whole choir put their collection in one small bag. This was dropped in turn into my bag by the basso-profundo on the extreme right of the lower row. I was told it was in bad taste to shake my bag in front of the soprano who never gave anything.

The Anglican Church in Dawson was heated by a huge drum-furnace in the basement. The heat opening was also large, about six feet square, placed directly above the drum and situated in front of the altar and covered by a grating. The heat was forced up by a powerful fan, activated by a thermostat in the church. One cold winter day Vance was celebrating a wedding in the church and, of course, the whole wedding-party stood on the grate. The ceremony had only just begun when the thermostat started the fan. The blast blew most of the women's skirts high over their heads—an embarrassing moment for the women but very entertaining for the men in the church!

Pungent paper-weight

Joe McCaffery, a prospector and trapper, came to me one day complaining that while he was urinating the stream was suddenly cut off, without any signal from him. An X-ray of his bladder showed a large stone about the size of a goose egg which was acting like a ball-valve. I distended his bladder with water to gain entry and then removed the stone through an incision in his abdomen. The surgery was successful and Joe boasted that his new, uninterrupted stream would "go over Ogilvie Bridge!", a span over the Klondyke River. The stone was brown and as hard as flint. I had it cut in half. The section showed attractive concentric rings of colour like an agate and I asked a jeweller to polish the cut surface so that I could use it as a paper-weight. But not for long. It had a persistent urinous odor so powerful that the cat stopped and sniffed when passing my desk. I had to throw it out!

EPILOGUE

Time to go

When the war was over it was time for me to leave the Yukon. The war had brought great changes to Dawson. At first Canada and the Allies needed to buy arms and supplies from the United States and gold was needed to help pay for them so Dawson's dredges worked day and night, full out. We lacked for nothing and the town's streets were full of people. But as soon as the Japanese attacked Pearl Harbor and the Americans became our allies the gold was not needed any more. The young men who had been working on the dredges were not needed any more, either, and left to join the army or to work in factories in Toronto, Winnipeg or Vancouver. My work-load, and pay, went down with a jolt, for I was paid on a per capita basis. And as the Americans moved to ward off any Japanese attacks on Alaska they began to send men and supplies from Seattle up the Inner Passage to Skagway. From Skagway they went by rail to Whitehorse and then down the Yukon to Alaska by steamer. Dawson, already diminished by the cuts in gold production, became merely a stopover for the crews and soldiers.

These changes meant that I was on my own again, the only doctor for hundreds of miles. I had been by myself in Mayo but then the death of my predecessor in Dawson from peritonitis (caused by tardily-treated appendicitis) made the authorities realise that a doctor could not work by himself. Two doctors would not only give better medical service but would also look after each other in case of illness. So when I arrived in Dawson I had been told to find an associate who could maintain the service to the hospital and to individual patients. I hired some young men who had helped me for months at a time while they got some money to continue their studies or to set themselves up in practice down south. Now that war had come to our part of the world I could not keep an assistant and he went off to join the army. After a few months of lonely work I decided to join the army myself. I was accepted by a board in Winnipeg but before I even got near a military patient Comptroller Jeckell telephoned the Minister of Defence and in short order I was out of the Army and back tending the sick in Dawson for nearly five years.

I finally decided to leave in 1947. The Yukon now had a fine medical service. The poverty that held back the territory during the Thirties was gone and equipment, drugs, facilities and doctors were in good supply. This was fine for the people but made life routine for me. If there was a difficult case I was now expected to refer the patient to a specialist in Whitehorse or to send them to Vancouver or Edmonton. There were fewer challenges and so I went to Edinburgh to sit for my Fellowship of the Royal College of Surgeons, returned to Canada and my family and began practice on the Prairies and then Vancouver. For a few years, however, I went back to the Yukon in the summer to do surgery and to relieve my brother, Dr. Barry Duncan.

What a life I had in the Yukon! I had more adventures in boats and planes than most people had in a life-time and had saved lives, tended the sick and brought hundreds of babies into the world. In my youth I dreamed of becoming a super-specialist with ultimate knowledge in a very limited field of academic medicine. This became impossible once I got into practice and I abandoned my goal of becoming, say, the Regius Professor of Omphaloscopy—the science of the observation of the belly-button!

However, now that the twilight is deepening, I realize that no better use of my limited talents could have been made than in the isolated environment of the sub-Arctic. It was a most satisfying experience; replete with adequate means, a good wife, a good family and many good friends.

APPENDIX

Those Little Houses

There is no direct relationship between the practice of medicine in the Yukon and the widespread use of outhouses in the Territory but it was hard to go on my daily rounds without hearing stories about these offices of easement built in windy backyards. Here are a few:

The Treadwell Yukon Company built a dilly of a biffy for the men who worked in the silver mine at Keno and one evening a miner decided it was the perfect spot in which to get rid of some gasoline-soaked rags. He had been fixing the transmission on his truck and wanted to leave everything nice and tidy. An hour or so later another miner came to the outhouse with a magazine under his arm and a package of cigarettes and some matches in his pocket. After a while, his task completed and his cigarette smoked down to the butt, he reached behind his back and threw the butt down the hole. The blast lifted him off the seat and soon he was in hospital being treated for burns to his buttocks. A friend came to cheer him up.

"Sorry to hear you got your ass burned, Pat. Hope you'll be better soon. We all miss you."

"Oh well," Pat replied, "it might have been worse. If I hadn't been thinking about my wife's sister, I would have lost everything !"

At another mining camp it was impossible to dig a hole for the outhouse because there was no soil, only solid granite. One of the firm's engineers, however, remembered that there was a steep cliff near the camp and he designed a cantilever structure that supported an outhouse projecting over the cliff for nearly six feet. Visitors to this outhouse could enjoy a marvellous view of the valley hundreds of feet below. But the engineer was obviously not an expert in aeronautics, for he forgot that cliffs create up-draughts. Many's the time toilet paper was returned to the embarrassed user. Some patrons were afraid of heights. For them going to this outhouse was like walking the plank with hundreds of feet of open space, not water, below. Others reported that the fear of falling worked better than castor oil. And the prospectors and trappers who walked along the trails below wondered how Eaton's managed to get such wide distribution for their catalogue.

Wise Yukoners used quite a few tricks to make their outhouses as comfortable as possible in winter. Some tacked rabbit fur to the rim of the hole to avoid frost-burn. Others used portable toilet seats that were kept warm by the kitchen stove. A thoughtful hostess always provided one for her guests. A small group of Yukoners, however, had no need for these devices. They were employees of the power companies and enjoyed free electricity. Two or three bulbs under the seat kept their bottoms warm. The big bosses of the power companies went even further and had electric heaters installed in their outhouses. Such luxury!

May your moccasins make happy tracks in the snow and the rainbow touch your shoulder!

ACKNOWLEDGMENTS

I want to thank the doctors who helped me in the last years of my practice in the Yukon: Dr. Geoff Homer, Dr. Frank Kells and especially my brother, Dr. Barry Duncan, who took over the Dawson practice. Thanks, also, to the Sisters of St. Anne for their help in Dawson, especially Sister Mary Faustina and Sister Mary Laurina. In Whitehorse I was grateful to Miss Florence McDonald and Miss Jean McTavish.

I remember with gratitude the work of the late Dr. Ed Hoodless and the late Dr. Jim Rennie and, of course, that of the late Mrs. Jean McCullum and the late Mrs. Jean Howatt.

My sincere thanks to my daughter-in-law, Candice Field, for typing and correcting my manuscript, to my step-son, Douglas Field, for processing some of the photographs used in the book, to Ted Ferguson and to Geoff Molyneux, who finally got the book to the printers.

I am grateful, too, for the help I have received from the people at Raincoast Books.